Infectious Disease Handbook for Emergency Care Personnel

Infectious Disease Handbook for Emergency Care Personnel

Katherine H. West, R.N., B.S.N., M.S. ED., C.I.C.

Infection Control Consultant
Emergency Medical Services Systems
Springfield, Virginia

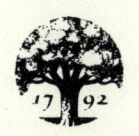

J. B. Lippincott Company   Philadelphia
London   Mexico City   New York   St. Louis
São Paulo   Sydney

Sponsoring Editor: Joyce Mkitarian
Production Editor: Carol Florence
Indexer: Sandra King
Design Director: Tracy Baldwin
Designer: Don Shenkle
Production Manager: Kathleen P. Dunn
Compositor: University Graphics, Inc.
Printer/Binder: R. R. Donnelley & Sons Co.

Copyright © 1987, by J. B. Lippincott Company. All rights reserved. No part of this book may be used or reproduced in any manner whatsoever without written permission except for brief quotations embodied in critical articles and reviews. Printed in the United States of America. For information write J. B. Lippincott Company, East Washington Square, Philadelphia, Pennsylvania 19105.

6 5 4 3 2 1

Library of Congress Cataloging-in-Publication Data

West, Katherine H.
    Infectious disease handbook for emergency care personnel.

    Includes bibliographies and index.
    1. Medical emergencies—Handbooks, manuals, etc.
2. Communicable diseases—Handbooks, manuals, etc.
3. Emergency medical personnel—Diseases and hygiene—Handbooks, manuals, etc.   I. Title.   [DNLM: 1. Communicable Diseases—handbooks.   2. Communicable Disease Control—handbooks.   3. Emergency Medical Services—handbooks. WC 39 W518i]
    RC86.8.W47   1987   614.4′4   86-10694
    ISBN 0-397-54611-4

This handbook is intended solely as a guide for the the appropriate procedures that are crucial when rendering emergency care. Since circumstances can vary from one emergency to another, this book is not intended as a statement of standards of care required in any particular situation. Also this book is not intended to legally advise emergency personnel concerning activities and procedures that are discussed. Such local determinations should be made with the aid of legal counsel. Nor is it intended that this Handbook shall in any way advise emergency personnel concerning legal authority to perform the activities or procedures discussed.

To Bruce

Whose guidance and support encouraged me to develop this contribution to the field of Emergency Medical Services

Contents

Introduction ix

1 Personal Health Concerns 1
    Establishing a Health Record 1
    Maintaining Immunizations 2
    Working When Ill 4
    Understanding the Formula for Infection 6

2 Avoiding Infection and Preventing Its Spread 9
    Recognizing Signs and Symptoms 9
    Handwashing Technique 11
    IV Site Preparation 13

3 Communicable Diseases 16
    Tuberculosis 16
    Hepatitis Viruses 19
    Meningitis 28
    Malaria (Jungle Fever) 31
    Rabies (Hydrophobia) 32
    Salmonella 34
    Impetigo 36
Childhood Diseases 37
    Measles 37
    Mumps (Infectious Parotitis) 40
    Chickenpox (Varicella Zoster) 40
    Pertussis (Whooping Cough) 42
Sexually Transmitted Diseases 44
    Gonorrhea 44
    Syphilis 45
    AIDS (Acquired Immune Deficiency Syndrome) 46

Cytomegalovirus Infection   50
Lice (Pediculosis)   51
Scabies   52

Herpes Viruses   52
Herpes Simplex (Types 1 and 2)   53
Herpes Zoster   60

4 Caring for Your Rescue Vehicle, Supplies, and Equipment   65

Recommendations for Cleaning Your Rescue Vehicle   65
Completing a Log Sheet   69
Disposal of Infectious Waste   70
Reusing Disposables   74
Cleaning and Maintaining Training Manikins   76
Supply Rotation   79
Stethoscopes   79
Multi-Dose Vials   79
Needle and Syringe Disposal   80
Respiratory Therapy Equipment   82
Antishock Trousers   86
IV Bags   87

5 Infection Control Program Costs   89

6 EMS–Hospital Relations: Establishing a Contact Person   92

Appendix   95
Infectious Disease Quick Reference   95
Glossary   103

Index   107

Introduction

Although the growth of emergency medical services (EMS) has been rapid in the past 10 years, organized emergency services have been in existence for over a century. In 1865 the United States Army formed the first ambulance service in an effort to reduce mortality rates during the Civil War. Hospital-based emergency services began in the 1940s in Cincinnati, Indianapolis, and New York.[1] Activities within these first emergency services, however, were limited to "scoop and haul." Advances were not made until 1966 when the Highway Safety Act was enacted. This act encouraged the expansion of EMS services across the nation.

In 1966 a study was released that captured national attention. This study, "Accidental Death and Disability: The Neglected Disease of Modern Society," emphasized the problem of prehospital mortality and revealed that billions of dollars were being spent on rehabilitating and supporting disabled accident victims.[2] Following the release of this study, recommendations were made for improving emergency medical services. In 1971 Congress held public hearings in various areas of the country to evaluate suggestions for EMS improvements. These hearings were conducted over a 3-year period and resulted in the enactment of the Emergency Medical Services Systems (EMSS) Act.[3] This act provided for personnel, facilities, and equipment for EMS systems formulation. EMS systems would supply emergency care to patients who had been victims of disasters or other emergency situations,[4] as well as provide care for nontrauma patients suffering from infections, communicable diseases, or chronic disease processes.

During the rapid growth of EMS, education in the areas of communicable diseases, infection processes, and health precautions for emergency personnel, as well as for patients, have not been addressed. EMS personnel have been concerned about these areas, however, and have asked many questions. Some of the questions most frequently asked include the following:

Who will notify me if I have been exposed to a patient with an infectious disease?
What can I do to protect myself when handling these patients?
What should I use to clean the vehicle?
What immunizations should I keep up-to-date?

The answers to these questions and many more could be incorporated into existing curricula. Informing EMS personnel about infectious, communicable, and chronic diseases would answer individual concerns, improve personnel skills, improve EMS in the community, and fulfill community expectations of the EMS system.[5]

This handbook will provide EMS personnel with quick reference sources that focus on situations involving infectious diseases and how to manage these diseases in the field. The main focus is what preventive measures EMS personnel can incorporate into their care to protect nontrauma patients and themselves.

Information is presented in categories listed in the Contents. For quick reference, begin in the Index to locate the page number for the specific information you need. The information is presented in an outline format for easy reference.

▌References

1. Barber J, Dillman P: *Emergency Patient Care for the EMT-A.* Norwalk, Reston Publishing, 1981
2. Accidental Death and Disability: The Neglected Disease of Modern Society, National Academy of Sciences, National Research Council, 1966
3. The United States Congressional Emergency Medical Services Systems Act of 1973, 93 USC, SB 2410
4. McKay JI: Historical review of emergency medical services, EMT roles, and EMT utilization in emergency departments. J Emer Nsg 11:27–32, 1985
5. Cross KP: Adults as Learners, pp 227–229. San Francisco, Jossey-Bass, 1981

Personal Health Concerns   1

When addressing personal health concerns of emergency medical services (EMS) personnel, two areas to consider are the health status of the care provider and the health status of the patient. Patients who are sick or injured are more susceptible to infection. Also, patients who may have communicable diseases might expose you to infection. Therefore, maintaining your health is important, not only for your own benefit, but also for the benefit of your patient.

A personal health maintenance program will help protect you and should include (1) personal hygiene education, (2) a system for monitoring work-related illnesses and exposures, (3) identification of work-related risks, and (4) development of policies and procedures for preventing risks.[1] This handbook will address each of these areas.

■ ESTABLISHING A PERSONAL HEALTH RECORD

The first area of importance is establishing a personal health record for yourself. Each member of the EMS, both paid and volunteer systems, should have a pre-employment physical examination. The physical examination can be performed by a physician, physician's assistant, or nurse practitioner and should include the following information and tests:

1. Communicable Disease History—It is important for you to record the diseases you have had and those you could still contract.
2. Chest X-Ray—A chest x-ray is necessary to establish a baseline and rule out any disease process present upon employment. This documents your health status when hired and shows any changes in your condition during the course of

employment that might be work related; this assists with compensation procedures.
3. TB Skin Test (purified protein derivative [PPD], *not* a tine test)—A tine test is a screening tool. As a member of a high-risk group, you should establish a more accurate baseline with a PPD.
4. Laboratory Tests
   a. VDRL (RPR)—This test for syphilis, designed by the Venereal Disease Research Laboratory, establishes a baseline.
   b. Hepatitis tests (HB_sAg and anti-HB_s)—Hepatitis screening is also required to establish baseline information and determines the need for possible immunization. This will be explained in detail in the section on hepatitis.[2]

■ MAINTAINING IMMUNIZATIONS

An immunization program is recommended for EMS personnel. The goals for such a program are preventing illnesses and handling complications that may accompany illnesses.[3]

It is important to keep your immunizations current as recommended below.

Tetanus–Diphtheria (Td) Vaccine—A booster for tetanus–diphtheria is required every 10 years. In 1981 the recommendation for tetanus toxoid immunization changed, the diphtheria vaccine was added to the tetanus immunization because the nation's population had not maintained immunization status against diphtheria. Since diphtheria primarily affects children, EMS personnel should maintain their levels of immunity if they are involved in child care.[4]

Many hospital emergency department personnel have not followed this recommendation of maintaining tetanus–diphtheria immunity. A study conducted by Brand and colleagues revealed that 23% of wound injuries were managed incorrectly, and 6% of wound injuries were undertreated.[5] The incidence of diphtheria in the United States is increasing: therefore, receiving recommended boosters is crucial.

Influenza (Flu) Vaccine—Although flu vaccines are optional, yearly inoculations should be encouraged to reduce personnel illness and patient exposure.

Each year epidemiologists predict the strains of flu that will dominate the flu season. Then vaccine is produced, usually containing three strains of virus. Receiving the vaccine on a yearly basis will build your immune status against a wide variety of viruses. Vaccination may also reduce personnel illness and absenteeism and will protect patients from unnecessary exposure.

Mumps Vaccine—Only a one-time injection of mumps vaccine is required. EMS personnel who have never had mumps may want to consider receiving this vaccine. Males especially need to consider being vaccinated, since 20% of adult males who contract mumps develop inflamed testes.[6]

Rubella Vaccine (German Measles)—Only a one-time injection of rubella vaccine is required. Rubella vaccine is a live virus vaccine and is recommended for all persons 12 months of age and older who are not immune. This vaccine is important especially for women of childbearing age,[7] although it is not recommended for pregnant women.

The primary goal of the worldwide immunization program is to reduce the incidence of rubella in preschool children and to prevent exposure of susceptible pregnant women. If a pregnant woman contracts rubella, the infant may be born with congential rubella syndrome (CRS). CRS may include multiple congenital anomalies and mental retardation. The ultimate goal is to eliminate CRS.

Hepatitis B Vaccine—A one-time series of three injections of hepatitis B vaccine is given over a 6-month period. This vaccine may require a booster 5 years after the initial series. The vaccine, Heptavax B, is recommended for all EMS personnel who are susceptible to hepatitis B. Studies conducted by Drs. Dienstag and Ryan have shown that emergency department nurses are at high risk for contracting hepatitis B because of their frequent contact with blood and secretions.[8] A study conducted by Dr. Craven and coworkers determined the risk of hepatitis B for prehospital care providers in the Boston area to be three times to five times greater than the risk to the general public.[9] Emergency medical personnel have been identified as a high-risk group and should be immunized.

The vaccine is administered in a series of three injections. An initial injection is followed by a second injection 4 weeks later, with the third injection given 6 months after the initial injection. Recent studies have revealed that some individuals require two additional injections to achieve full immunity. An antibody level should be ascertained after the initial series of injections to document immunity.[10]

Concerns regarding the safety of the hepatitis vaccine were addressed in a series of studies published in December, 1984. The main concern was the possiblity of transmitting acquired immune deficiency syndorme (AIDS), but in a series of controlled tests, the refining process for the hepatitis vaccine was shown to kill the AIDS agent.[11] The hepatitis vaccine is considered to be one of the safest vaccines produced.

■ WORKING WHEN ILL

Another health concern you may have is whether to work or to stay home when you are ill. Working when you are ill poses an additional risk to patients as well as to your coworkers. Contracting viruses or infections from you may create serious problems for compromised patients. When should you stay home? Here are some brief guidelines to help you decide:

Disease or Condition	Work Status
Positive PPD skin test	May work with followup x-ray or medication. Remember, a positive test does not mean you have tuberculosis; it means you have been exposed.
Conjunctivitis (infectious)	May work, but with no patient contact until drainage subsides. Good handwashing technique is essential.
Diarrhea	Do not work until symptoms subside or the stool culture for infection is negative.

Draining wound	Do not work until culture is negative. Wound should be dressed.
Herpes simplex (cold sore)	May work, but no contact with high-risk (immunocompromised) patients until your lesions are dry and crusted.
Herpes zoster (shingles)	May work with lesions covered, but no contact with high-risk (immunosuppressed) patients.
Herpetic whitlow (hands or fingers)	Do not work until lesions heal, because it is not known whether gloves prevent transmission.
Hepatitis A	Do not work until 7 days after jaundice appears and you have received medical clearance.
Hepatitis B	Wear gloves when you are in contact with a patient's mucous membranes or nonintact skin until you have received medical clearance.
Mononucleosis (mono)	Do not work until all symptoms have subsided.
Lice or scabies	Do not work until you have been treated with an appropriate lotion or shampoo.
Strep infection	Do not work until you have taken prescribed drugs for 24 hours.
Measles	Do not work until 7 days after rash appears.
Mumps	Do not work until 9 days after glands began to enlarge.
Chickenpox	Do not work until lesions are completely crusted and dried.
Upper respiratory infection or flu	May work, but no contact with high-risk patients until your symptoms subside.
Impetigo	May work, but no patient contact until crusts heal.[1]

Developing EMS Systems Policies

Another aspect of working or not working when ill includes developing policies to follow personnel who have been exposed to infections or communicable diseases. Ideally, these policies should encourage EMS personnel to report exposures without penalty. If an employee feels he will have to use his sick leave or take leave without pay, there may be poor compliance with the program.

Policy development should address work-related and non-work-related exposures. Because work-related illnesses will be covered by Workers' Compensation, policy development should focus on approaches to cover incubation periods and non-work-related exposures in order to reduce risks for all personnel and patients.[8]

■ UNDERSTANDING THE FORMULA FOR INFECTION

To better understand why and when you are at risk of infection, study the following formula:

$$\text{Infection} = \frac{\text{Dose} \times \text{virulence}}{\text{Resistance of host}}$$

Dose = the number of viable (live) organisms present to cause infection.

Virulence = strength or ability of bacteria or virus to infect.

Resistance of host = an interruption in the body's normal defense mechanism, which allows the organism to enter the body (e.g., an open sore or break in the skin or in mucous membranes).

Each of the above factors must be present for infection to occur. When you suspect exposure to an infection or communicable disease, apply this formula with the three factors. This process may help you decide if you need further evaluation.

If you are screened after exposure to an infectious or communicable disease, questions will be asked in an attempt to work out this infection formula. Therefore, it is important that you answer the questions in a factual and honest manner. Working out this formula will help differentiate actual risks from perceived risks. Although you will not know the specific number of bacteria or virus present, you will know whether you were in contact with a small amount or large amount of blood or body fluid.

For example, you have transported an infant with a fever and rash. Later you are advised that the child has meningitis. What is your risk? Now apply the formula.

1. Dose—The causative organism for meningitis lives in nasopharyngeal secretions. Were you in direct contact with a small amount or a large amount of these secretions?
2. Virulence—Organisms causing bacterial meningitis are not able to survive long when exposed to air and light.
3. Resistance—How would these bacteria have entered your body? Did you give CPR? Did you suction the infant? Did the infant cough in your face? If the answer to all three questions is no, you are not considered at risk. If the answer to one of the three questions is yes, then some degree of risk is present, and you should contact your medical director. Also to be considered is your health status. Are you in good health, or are you working with a viral infection and reduced ability to combat an illness? If you are in good health, the risk is diminished.

■ References

1. Williams WW: CDC guidelines for infection control in hospital personnel. Infect Control 4:329–331; 346–347, 1983
2. Werdegar D: Guidelines for infection control aspects of employee health. APIC Journal September: 17–22, 1977
3. Wiederman G et al: Risk and benefits of vaccinations. Infect Control 5:438–444, 1984
4. Immunization Practice Advisory Committee: Diphtheria, tetanus and pertussis vaccine. MMWR 30:392–405, 1981
5. Brand DA et al: Adequacy of antitetanus prophylaxis in six hospital emergency rooms. N Engl J Med 309:636–640, 1983
6. The Merck Manual of Diagnosis and Therapy, 11th ed, pp. 742–745. Merck, Sharp & Dohme Research Laboratories, 1966
7. Rubella Prevention. Epidemiol Bulletin 84, No. 10:1984

8. Dienstag JL Ryan DM: Occupational exposure to hepatitis B virus in hospital personnel: Infection or immunization? Am J Epidemiol 115:26-39, 1982
9. Craven DE et al: Hepatitis B exposure in emergency medical personnel. Am J Med 75:269-272, 1983
10. Suboptimal response to hepatitis B vaccine given by injection into the buttock. MMWR 34:105-108, 1985
11. Hepatitis B vaccine: Evidence confirming lack of AIDS transmission. MMWR 33:685-687, 1984

Avoiding Infection and Preventing Its Spread   2

Two important methods of preventing unnecessary exposure to communicable diseases are recognizing signs and symptoms of infection and implementing protective measures. In field situations, you are working without the benefit of diagnoses. Therefore, the best approach may be to use those methods suggested by the signs and symptoms that patients present and to consider all body fluids as contaminated. In addition, incorporating a thorough handwashing technique into your routine will help you avoid contamination and infection, and properly preparing the site of IV needle insertion helps protect your patients.

■ RECOGNIZING SIGNS AND SYMPTOMS

When caring for your patients, watch for the following presenting signs and symptoms and follow the recommended preventive measures.

Rash and Fever of Unknown Origin

The patient who presents with fever and a rash may have a communicable disease that could be spread through contact with oral or respiratory secretions. Therefore, your preventive measure should be to use a mask and, if possible, the patient should be the one to wear the mask. Using masks will help stop the spread of organisms at the site. If the patient is uncooperative, however, just mask yourself.

Diarrhea

When the patient presents with diarrhea, he could have an infection, such as *Salmonella* or *Shigella*. These organisms can be spread through the stools. In this situation, your preventive measures are to use a good handwashing technique and to wear disposable gloves, if possible.

Draining Wounds

Infection may be present in a patient with a draining wound, especially if the wound is surrounded by a reddened area. Wounds are generally infected with organisms that do not spread through the air. Therefore, your preventive measures are to wear disposable gloves and to use a thorough handwashing technique.

Jaundice

Jaundice may or may not be infectious. Jaundice indicates the presence of several different illnesses and does not always mean the patient has hepatitis. However, be cautious and protect yourself by wearing disposable gloves and using a thorough handwashing technique.

Dialysis Patients

Although dialysis is not a sign or a symptom, it is important to discuss it here because you may encounter a patient with a peritoneal catheter in place (Fig. 2-1). By being able to recognize this catheter and what it indicates, you can take precatuions against possible infection.

The patient with a history of renal failure who is on hemodialysis or peritoneal dialysis should be considered a candidate for hepatitis B. Studies have shown that these patients have high incidences of hepatitis B. Also, peritoneal dialysis patients are susceptible to peritonitis and will require hospital care. Be careful when handling blood and secretions from these patients.

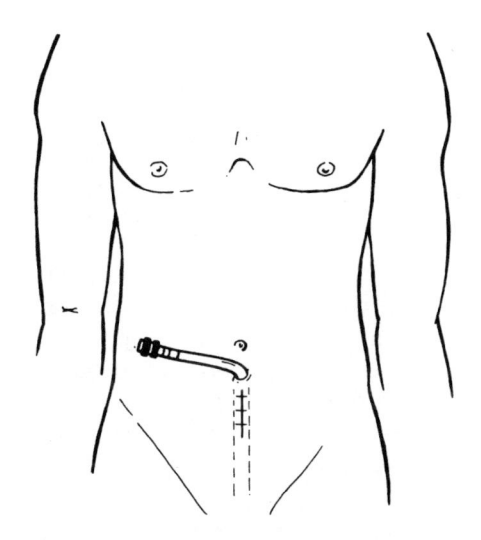

Figure 2-1. A patient receiving peritoneal dialysis may be in a high-risk group for hepatitis B. Use caution when handling the catheter drainage.

Your preventive measures are to wear disposable gloves and to use a thorough handwashing technique.

Some EMS systems have set up kits for their vehicles that contain essential supplies such as disposable gloves, masks, and plastic bags for disposing of infected secretions or waste.

■ HANDWASHING TECHNIQUE

If one were to ask, "What is the *one* measure that would offer the best protection in the field?" the answer would be—handwashing. However, although thorough handwashing technique is the single *most* effective preventive measure for medical personnel in the field, good handwashing procedures often are not practiced by members of health care teams. Researchers have concluded that, although handwashing technique is usually part of practical and theoretical health care curricula, medical personnel only use appropriate handwashing procedures about 30% of the time. Studies also have indicated that, although thorough handwashing is important to prevent infection from spreading to patients, medical personnel reported they were too busy to perform the procedure.[1]

In field situations, running water for handwashing is not always available. However, several products on the market can be used without water, such as Hibistat, Alcare, and Cal-stat.[2] Because these products are alcohol based, when you apply one of the solutions to your hands and rub them together, friction will cause the solution to evaporate, killing surface organisms. Using one of these solutions is a temporary preventive measure until you are able to perform a more thorough handwashing technique. Plain soap and water are adequate for routine handwashing, but for high-risk and invasive procedures, use an antiseptic solution.

Proper handwashing includes the following steps:

1. Use an acceptable soap (see Table 2-1).
2. Work up a lather, using friction for 15 seconds.
3. Rinse hands well and dry them with a paper towel.
4. Important—use a paper towel to turn off the faucet.

A review of handwashing agents is presented in Table 2-1.

Table 2-1. REVIEWING HANDWASHING AGENTS

Handwashing Agents	Brand Names	Action
Bar soaps	Safeguard Ivory Dial	Helps remove organisms, but doesn't kill them.
Liquid soap antiseptic	Safe 'N Sure Kindness Kare	Helps remove organisms, but doesn't kill them.
Alcohol foam agents	Alcare Cal-stat	Kills staph, strep, and fungus organisms.
Povidone–iodine	Betadine Acu-dyne Prepadyne	Kills staph, strep, and fungus organisms.
Chlorhexidine gluconate	Hibiclens Hibistat	Kills staph, strep, fungus, and viruses.

■ IV SITE PREPARATION

Preparation of the IV site prior to introducing the needle or catheter is of vital importance ... to the patient.

Unfortunately, often short cuts are taken. It is important to remember that entry into the venous system creates a direct pathway for bacteria to enter the system. Conducting a proper site prep, whevever possible, gives your patient an added measure of protection against acquisition of a bloodstream infection.

Which solution is most appropriate? Table 2-2 lists the recommended solutions established by the Centers for Disease Control (CDC). The first method recommended is 2% tincture of iodine, followed by alcohol. This is the most effective method, but it is a two-step procedure that is not practical in the field situation.

The second recommended solution is a povidone–iodine combination. This solution is chemically different from tincture of iodine and is not followed by alcohol. Thus, this is a one-step procedure that affords your patient a good level of protection. If the patient states that he or she is iodine allergic, ascertain what reaction is incurred. In the case of true iodine allergy, alcohol may be substituted. However, to be of benefit alcohol needs to be applied as a 30-second friction rub, which is time consuming and not as effective as a povidone–iodine solution.

Solutions should be applied as shown in Figure 2-2. Using a circular motion, begin in the center and work outward. Never return to the center.

The application of ointments following needle or catheter insertion varies in different areas of the country. Generally, for field lines it is not necessary to place an ointment at the insertion site, because usually circumstances are far from ideal, and debris may become mixed with the ointment.[3]

Another important aspect in prevention of infection or irritation at the insertion site is stabilization of the needle or catheter hub. The method most frequently recommended in the literature is the "chevron" method, which involves the use of a criss-cross technique. A long, ¼" piece of tape is placed under the needle or catheter hub. Then each end of the tape is crossed over to the opposite side and secured to the patient's skin.[4]

Table 2-2. IV SITE PREP RECOMMENDATIONS

Antiseptic	Advantages	Disadvantages	Special Considerations
Iodine solution 2%, tincture 2%	Kills bacteria, fungi viruses, protozoa, and yeasts Inexpensive and reliable	May burn or chap skin May cause an allergic reaction Discolors skin	Always ask the patient if he has any allergies before applying. Wash off the iodine with 70% alcohol after 30 seconds. Don't cover the skin before the iodine is washed off. Never mix iodine with hydrogen peroxide.
Povidone–iodine (water-soluble complexes of iodine and organic compounds; also called iodophors) Betadine, Proviodine, Sepp	Less irritating than iodine tinctures or solutions Doesn't stain skin as much as iodine	Less effective than regular iodine solutions May be absorbed through the skin during prolonged use May cause an allergic reaction	Always ask the patient if he has any alergies before applying. Do not wash it off—use full strength.

(West KH: Infection control and IV therapy. JORRI III (8):14–17, 1983)

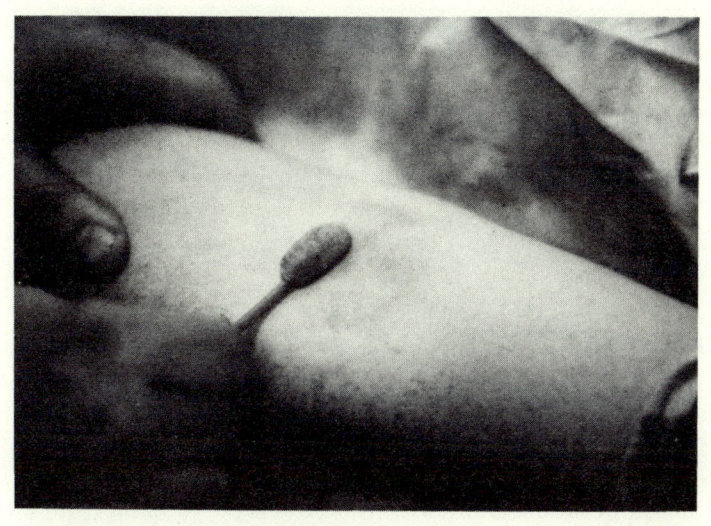

Figure 2-2. Applying antiseptic.

References

1. Larson E, Killien M: Factors influencing handwashing behavior of patient care personnel. Am J Infect Control 10:3:93–99, 1982
2. Handwashing alternatives. Hospital Infect Control 35, March 1977
3. Strom J, Hill WI: Prehospital IV administration: And some considerations. J Emerg Nursing May–June, 4(3):24–25, 1978
4. Nursing Photobook: Managing IV Therapy, p. 37. Horsham, Intermed Communications, 1980

Communicable Diseases 3

■ TUBERCULOSIS

Tuberculosis (TB) is not a highly communicable disease. It is a disease that still occurs in the United States population, but not as frequently as it occurred 30 or 40 years ago when living conditions and personal habits were below today's standards.[1]

In 1982, 25,000 cases of TB were diagnosed in the United States. The incidence of TB in this country had been declining at the rate of 5% per year until 1975, when the rate of decline dropped to only 1.4% per year. The reason for the change was the influx of Indo-Chinese refugees into this country.[2]

In 1985, TB began to decline again in the United States. Intense screening programs and new drug therapy regimens have had a significant effect on this recent decline. Also, more and more information is available about the disease process and transmission.

TB is usually acquired early in life and does not cause illness until the person is over 45 years of age. Then the patient may develop a chronic illness or a change in immune status, resulting in reactivation of TB disease. The incidence of TB is highest in males and in nonwhite populations.[3]

The causative organism for pulmonary TB is *Mycobacterium tuberculosis*, which is spread by droplets from an infected patient. Droplets are created when an infected individual coughs, sneezes, or sings. If you inhale these droplets, you could contract TB. It is felt, however, that prolonged contact with an infected patient usually is necessary to place you at risk.[4] Prolonged contact is defined as living or working with an infected individual, so that transporting one would not place you at high risk. If the patient coughs, sneezes, or requires suctioning, intubation, or mouth-to-mouth ventilations, the degree of risk increases but still remains small.

The patient with TB may present with signs and symptoms such as productive cough, fever with profuse night sweats, unexplained weight loss, weakness, and hemoptysis (coughing up blood).[5] As these symptoms may suggest other medical problems, confirmation of a positive TB diagnosis may take time. Also, there are many types of TB, and not all of them are communicable. Therefore, specific tests need to be conducted. For example, a culture report may take 3 weeks to 6 weeks to yield a definite result. Meanwhile, you should be informed of any possible risks, depending on the care you gave the patient. Figure 3-1 illustrates the procedure used to screen patients and patient contacts and demonstrates the importance of the screening and testing processes.

Infectious agent: Mycobacterium tuberculosis.
Mode of transmission: Airborne droplets, primarily during sneezing, coughing, speaking, or singing.[2] Prolonged contact with an active TB case is most significant, as is contact with thick, coughed-up sputum.
Incubation period: 4 weeks to 12 weeks.
Symptoms: Cough, fever, night sweats, weight loss, fatigue, and hemoptysis (coughing up blood).[3]
Protective measures: Mask the patient, if possible, If not possible, mask yourself. Rapid fresh air ventilation, as available in your vehicle.
Followup for exposure: Necessary only if protective measures are not taken. Document exposure on your incident report form.
　1. PPD skin test or chest x-ray following contact, if not documented when you were hired. PPD should be given as soon as possible after contact and should be repeated in 6 weeks. If previously tested, you should have a PPD 6 weeks following the exposure.
　2. Repeat PPD or chest film 2 months to 3 months after the exposure.
　3. If your previous skin test was negative, and it is positive following the exposure, this could mean that
　　a. The TB organism is present in your body but is not causing disease.

18 ■ COMMUNICABLE DISEASES

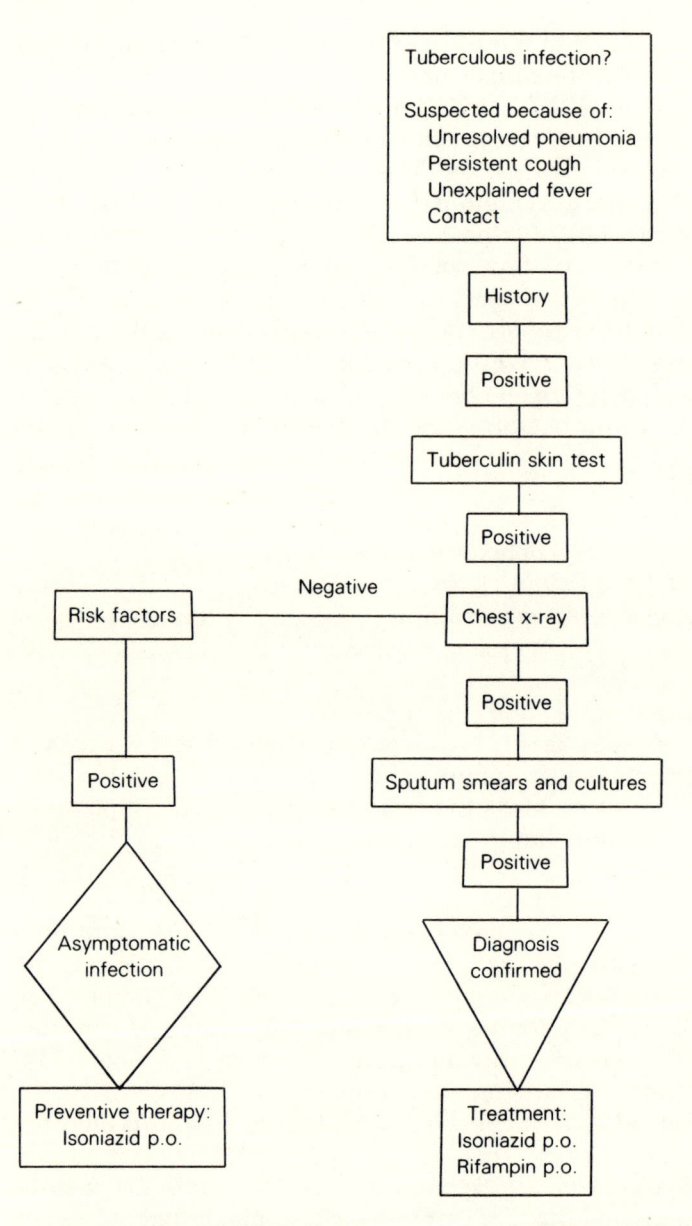

Figure 3-1. Screening and testing process when tuberculosis infection is suspected. (Adapted from Daniel TM, Mahmoud AAF, Warren KS: Algorithms in the diagnosis of and management of exotic diseases, XVI: Tuberculosis. J Infec Dis 134: 417–421, 1976)

b. You may be given a drug called Isoniazid (INH) to take for 1 year. If you are over 35 years old, INH may not be recommended as it has been associated with drug-induced hepatitis[3] in this age group.

■ HEPATITIS VIRUSES

Hepatitis is an inflammation of the liver that can be caused by a virus, alcohol consumption, or drug therapy. However, not all types of hepatitis are communicable. The only types that can be transmitted are those caused by viruses, and each type is spread in a specific manner.

The communicable forms of hepatitis are hepatitis A, hepatitis B, delta agent, and non-A, non-B hepatitis. Symptoms for all types of hepatitis are the same regardless of the cause. The initial symptoms are lowgrade fever, headache, loss of appetite, nausea, diarrhea and, occasionally, right upper quadrant pain. When the patient enters the second phase of illness, jaundice develops, urine turns dark brown, and stools become clay colored.

Hepatitis A (Viral)

Hepatitis A is most commonly referred to as viral or infectious hepatitis. This disease usually follows oral ingestion of the virus. Common sources include contaminated food or drinking water. Hepatitis A is very common in children, and most children who have hepatitis A are asymptomatic; they can, however, transmit infection to family members or other children with whom they have close daily contact.

INCUBATION PERIOD

The incubation period for hepatitis A is relatively short, 2 weeks to 6 weeks. Most of the virus is shed in stool. The virus is present in the blood of infected patients, but only for a short time. Once jaundice appears, the patient is no longer shedding virus.

DIAGNOSIS

Diagnosing viral hepatitis requires performing a hepatitis A viral test (HAV) and evaluating the presence of immunity. This test consists of two immune blood studies, an IgM, which shows current infection, and an IgG, which reveals previous infection.

Hepatitis A usually is uncomplicated, and the patient develops antibodies. There have been no documented cases of people developing chronic infection or becoming carriers of hepatitis A, therefore, it can be described as a mild disease.

Infectious agent: Hepatitis A virus
Mode of transmission: Contact with stool, blood, or urine of an infected person
Incubation period: 25 days to 30 days
Symptoms: Fever, weakness, loss of appetite, nausea, abdominal pain; later, jaundice, dark colored urine, light colored stools.
Protective measures: Handwashing following contact with excretions, or using disposable gloves.
Followup for exposure: Necessary only if protective measures were not used. Usually immunization with immune serum globulin (ISG) as soon as possible after exposure.[7]

Hepatitis B (Serum)

Hepatitis B is commonly referred to as serum hepatitis and is associated with the use of contaminated drug paraphernalia. This virus is found in the liver and blood of infected patients. Hepatitis B virus can be transmitted through contact with secretions from the oral cavity or genital tract of an infected patient. In fact, hepatitis B now is listed as a sexually transmitted disease. Transmission can occur also by using contaminated razors and toothbrushes, and an infected mother can transmit infection to her fetus through the placenta.

INCUBATION PERIOD

The incubation period for hepatitis B is quite long, up to 200 days after exposure, which can make identification of a specific contact very difficult. In fact, most patients with hepatitis B do not have a clear history of exposure.

SYMPTOMS

As mentioned previously, the symptoms are the same for all types of hepatitis. However, the initial, or flulike, symptoms of serum hepatitis are often the only symptons the patient experiences. Therefore, many cases of serum hepatitis are passed off as cases of flu and are never positively identified as hepatitis. Laboratory tests are available, however, to evaluate all phases of hepatitis B infections.

INTERPRETING HEPATITIS B LABORATORY TESTS

Understanding hepatitis laboratory tests is difficult. It is important, however, that you become familiar with the tests and their meanings for your own benefit. If you are involved in the care of a patient who is being tested for hepatitis B, follow up on the lab test results. Table 3-1 and the test descriptions that follow are presented to help you understand the lab tests and to explain what each test or combination of tests means.

HB_sAg (Hepatitis B Surface Antigen). When this test is reported as positive, or reactive, the patient is considered infectious. If the test remains reactive or positive for longer than 6 months, the patient is considered a "carrier."

Table 3-1. INTERPRETING SERUM HEPATITIS TESTS

HB_sAg	anti-HB_c	anti-HB_s	Interpretation
−	−	−	Susceptible, never had hepatitis B
+	−	−	Currently infected with hepatitis B virus.
+	+	−	Acute case or chronic carrier.
+	−	+	Potentially infectious.
+	+	+	
−	+	−	Transient state found in convalescent period of Hepatitis B.
−	+	+	Immune. Previous infection with (or immunization against) HBV, not infectious.
−	−	+	

(West KH: The dilemma—hepatitis B: What is it all about? JORRI, December 1982)

Anti-HB$_s$ (Antibody to HB$_s$Ag). The presence of an antibody level following hepatitis indicates convalescence. When this level is measured following vaccine administration, it verifies immunity.

Anti-HB$_c$ (Antibody to Hepatitis B Core Antigen). This level can usually be detected as soon as clinical disease becomes evident and remains present as long as the hepatitis B virus is multiplying. When the disease has resolved, the antibody level decreases but remains detectable for the life of the patient. This test is important during a phase of the disease called the "window phase," during which the HB$_s$Ag level declines and there is not sufficient antibody level for detection. If these two tests are the only tests performed, it may appear that the patient does not have hepatitis B. However, the anti-HB$_c$ is detectable and is a clue to previous hepatitis B disease.

Each test alone provides little information; performed together, these tests can support a diagnosis.[8,9]

Screening tests such as these have shown that a higher incidence of chronic illness occurs in patients who contract hepatitis B infections and only present flulike symptoms. Of these patients, it is estimated that 10% will probably become carriers, and 3% to 5% will probably develop chronic active hepatitis, with a greater risk of developing liver cancer. Thus, hepatitis B is different from hepatitis A not only because it is caused by a different virus, but because hepatitis B can have long-term effects for many patients who acquire it.

There is no treatment or cure for hepatitis B. Preventive measures include receiving Heptavax B (hepatitis B vaccine), wearing disposable gloves when possible, and using a thorough handwashing technique.

A study conducted at Massachusetts General Hospital by Dienstag and Ryan[10] showed that health care workers were at greater risk for contracting hepatitis B than the general population. Recently a group in Boston City[11] studied the incidence of hepatitis B in prehospital care providers. Their study showed that of the 87 participants, 18% has positive antibody markers for hepatitis B. They estimated that EMS personnel had a three to five times greater risk of developing hepatitis B infection than the general public and have recommended immunization of EMS personnel with the hepatitis B vaccine.

Infections agent: Hepatitis B virus
Mode of transmission: Blood, mucous membranes (saliva, sputum), sexual contact
Incubation period: 42 days to 200 days.
Symptoms: Nausea, loss of appetite, fatigue, abdominal pain, diarrhea, jaundice.
Protective measures: Wear disposable gloves when in contact with blood, saliva, or sputum. Use good handwashing technique.

Delta Agent

Delta agent is a newly identified hepatitis virus. In many ways it is a pseudovirus because it requires the presence of the hepatitis B virus to act as a host. In other words, the delta agent "piggybacks" the hepatitis B virus. When combined with the heptitis B virus, the delta agent often results in fulminant, or rapidly progressive, hepatitis.

The delta agent can be isolated from liver tissue but is not readily isolated from blood. Drug addicts have the greatest risk for delta agent infection. Hepatitis B carriers are more at risk than noncarriers. Laboratory tests are now available to test for delta agent, and delta agent research will continue.[12,13]

Non-A, Non-B Hepatitis

Non-A, non-B hepatitis (NANB) is a new form of hepatitis. This form was recognized when patients with acute and chronic hepatitis were tested for hepatitis A and hepatitis B, but neither form of hepatitis was identified as the cause of the illness. Many researchers feel that more than one virus may be responsible. There are no laboratory tests available to identify non-A, non-B hepatitis; diagnosis is made by elimination of hepatitis A or hepatitis B diseases.

Non-A, non-B hepatitis appears to be associated with transfusion illness. Typically, the patient begins to feel ill 6 weeks to

8 weeks following a transfusion and complains of fatigue and loss of appetite. Usually jaundice does not appear, but chronic illness results in 30% to 40% of the cases. This form of hepatitis parallels hepatitis B in many ways, but is not caused by the same virus.

Treating Needle-Stick Injuries

Needle-stick injuries should not be disregarded. Contaminated needles can transfer diseases such as hepatitis B and non-A, non-B hepatitis from the blood of an infected patient. If you receive a needle-stick injury, followup treatment is recommended. The specific treatment for such injuries depends on (1) the patient's availability for testing, (2) the results of the patient's blood screening report for hepatitis B, (3) the results of your blood screening report for hepatitis B, and (4) the patient's liver function studies.

UNKNOWN SOURCE

You may not know which patient was in contact with the needle before you were injured. For example, if you were cleaning out the drug box and were stuck by a needle someone had thrown in the box, you would have no way of knowing who had been treated with that particular needle. You still need to be treated. First, complete an incident report to document what happened. Second, seek treatment in a hospital emergency department, Public Health Department, or a physician's office.

The protocol for treating a needle-stick injury from an unknown source is demonstrated in Figure 3-2. Usually immune serum globulin (ISG) is administered. The dose is calculated according to the recommended dose of 0.6 ml/kg of body weight. ISG is administered to protect you against non-A, non-B hepatitis. You also need the initial injection of Heptavax B (hepatitis B vaccine), followed by two additional injections to complete the series. Before receiving the vaccine, your blood will be drawn and tested for HB_sAB (hepatitis B surface antibody). This test will indicate any immunity you may already have. If you are immune you will not need the vaccine.[7,14,15] Some protocols recommend liver function studies 6 months after the initial evaluation. This may vary from one area of the country to another.

```
                    ↓                              ↓
              Source unknown                  Source known
                    |                              |
                    ↓                              ↓
                   ISG                        Patient chart
              Heptavax if                      checked
              employee is           ╱              |
              HB Ab ⊖        Normal liver          ↓
                    |        function and    Elevated liver enzymes
                    ↓        HB Ag           ISG for employee
                 6-mo              |                |
              evaluation           ↓                ↓
                             No treatment      Check HB Ag of
                             to employee         patient
                                        ⊖    ╱         ╲ ⊕
                                       ╱               ╲
                                  No further          Ck employee
                                  treatment           HB₅Ab ⊖
                                                ⊕         |
                                               No         ↓
                                            treatment  HBIG 0.06 ml/kg
                                                          &
                                                       Heptavax
                                                          |
                                                          ↓
                                                        6-mo
                                                     evaluation
```

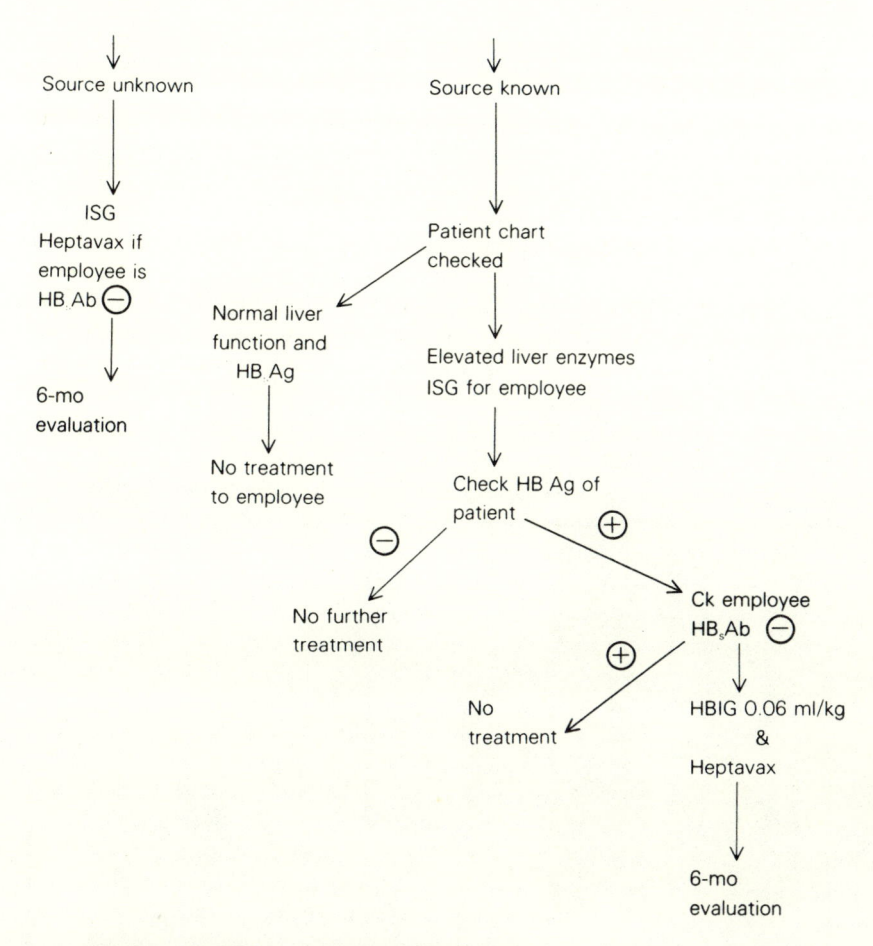

Figure 3-2. Needle-stick followup protocol.

KNOWN SOURCE

Figure 3-2 also outlines the protocol for a needle-stick injury from a known source. In most situations, you will know who the patient is. For example, you were starting an intravenous injection (IV), the patient pulled away, and you stuck yourself with the needle. First, the patient's liver will be evaluated through liver function studies, and he will also be checked for hepatitis B. If the serum glutamic-oxaloacetic transaminase (SGOT) is greater than 100, you will need ISG to protect you against non-

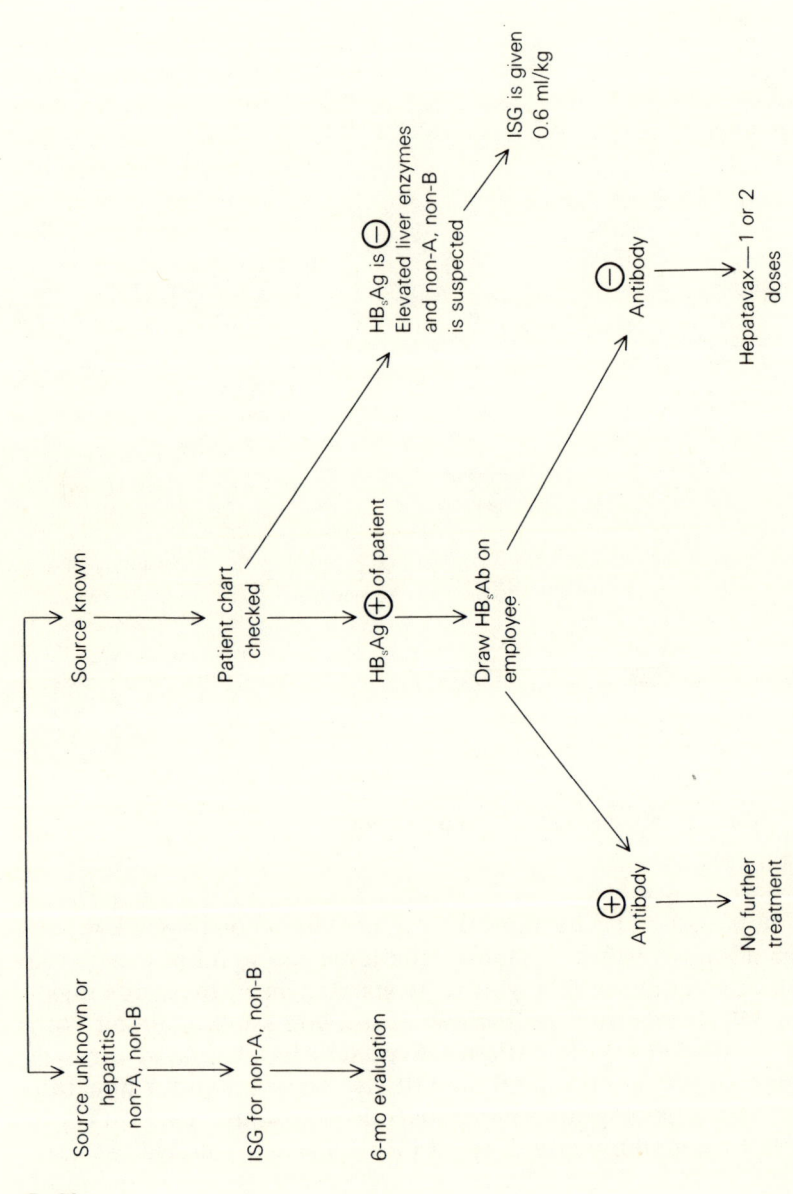

Figure 3-3. Postvaccine needle-stick protocol.

A, non-B hepatitis. If the SGOT and the HB_sAg are normal, you will require no further treatment. However, if the patient's HB_sAg is reactive you should receive more treatment.

The next step would be to check your HB_sAb (hepatitis B surface antibody). Since antibodies indicate immunity, if this test is negative or nonreactive you will need to receive HBIG (hepatitis B immune globulin). This globulin is specific for hepatitis B and is given in a dose of 0.06 ml/kg of body weight. New data suggest that the hepatitis B vaccine also administered at this time will provide prolonged immunity. Administration of HBIG alone has been shown to be only 75% effective and only provides temporary protection.[10] If you receive the vaccine, remember to schedule two additional injections to complete the series. The deltoid muscle is the recommended injection site. The second injection of the vaccine will be 4 weeks after the first injection, and the last injection will be 6 months after the first injection. All three injections are essential for effective treatment results.[7,11]

The hepatitis B vaccine has been found to be very effective and offers protection for a 4-year to 5-year period before a booster would be required. However, recent data have revealed that some individuals do not develop antibodies after the initial vaccine series. Desired antibody (immunity) level is achieved after two additional vaccine shots. In other words, beware of a false sense of security should you suffer subsequent needle-stick injuries after your vaccine series.

Postvaccine antibody levels should be measured and verified, and a protocol for postvaccine needle-stick injuries should be developed and followed. Figure 3-3 briefly describes the protocol for a needle-stick injury after the vaccine has been administered. If the source is unknown, ISG should be given to protect against non-A, non-B hepatitis. A 6-month evaluation is recommended.

Figure 3-3 also illustrates the postvaccine protocol when the source is known. The patient's chart is checked, and a blood sample is drawn. If the patient is positive for hepatitis B, your antibody level should be checked to verify immunity. If you have developed antibodies, no booster shot is necessary. If the patient's SGOT liver study is elevated, and the patient is suspected of having non-A, non-B hepatitis (a history of recent transfusions), ISG will be given to you in the recommended dosage.

Because the incidence of hepatitis B may be lower in some areas of the country, protocols may vary somewhat. Be aware of the protocols in the area where you work. All costs involved in needle-stick followup are covered under Workers' Compensation and should not render an expense to you, your service, or the hospital.

Summary: Exposure Follow-Up for Needle Stick

1. Document exposure.
2. Immune serum globulin (ISG) will be given and blood studies performed on you and the patient to determine presence of disease, immunity, or nonimmunity. HB_sAg (hepatitis B surface antigen) and anti-HB_s (antibody) lab studies will be performed.
3. If the patient is positive for hepatitis B, you should receive hepatitis B immune globulin (HBIG), which is given as one injection. Hepatitis B vaccine should also be given, as a series: the initial injection, another injection 4 weeks later, and the third injection 6 months after the first injection.
4. If you are negative for hepatitis B and the patient cannot be located, you should recieve ISG. The dosage will be calculated according to your body weight.
5. If both you and the patient are negative for hepatitis B, ISG is the only immunization you need. (see page 24 for further information).

■ MENINGITIS

Meningitis is an inflammation of the membrane linings that cover the brain and spinal cord. EMS personnel are often alarmed about meningitis because it has been considered a highly communicable disease. As with some other diseases discussed in this handbook, however, the mode of transmission is specific, and the risk to emergency care personnel is minimal.

Basically, there are two types of meningitis, the type caused by a specific bacteria and the type caused by a virus. Each type has an important difference with regard to communicability.

Bacterial Meningitis

Bacterial meningitis is caused by specific bacteria. Infection occurs when bacteria invade the subarachnoid space (the space in the brain between the arachnoid and the pia mater). This bacterial invasion extends into linings to the brain, entering the body through the bloodstream. Almost any bacteria may gain access through the bloodstream and cause illness,[16] but the most common bacteria causing meningitis are *Neisseria meningitidis, Haemophilus influenzae, Streptococcus pneumoniae,* and *E coli*.[17]

Bacterial meningitis commonly affects young children, especially children less than 1 year old. This type of meningitis is uncommon in adults over 25 years old and rare in adults over 40 years old.[16,18] Young children are at a greater risk because they are exposed to bacteria during the birth process. Meningococcal meningitis creates the greatest concern, although this type is not highly communicable, as was once thought.

The organism that causes meningococcal meningitis is *Neisseria meningitidis*, which lives in the nasopharynx. No other source has been identified. Some people are asymptomatic carriers and, since studies indicate that this organism may take weeks to spread among household members, transmission is probably the result of direct contact with nasopharyngeal secretions. Kissing, for example, or close contact when a child is coughing, could result in transmission.

SIGNS AND SYMPTOMS

The onset of signs and symptoms is rapid and usually follows a respiratory illness.[19] The most common signs and symptoms include fever, nausea, stiff neck, headache, vomiting, and a rash that appears on the lower trunk of the body.[16,17]

DIAGNOSIS

The initial diagnosis of meningitis is made on the basis of signs and symptoms. Next, a gram stain is performed on cerebrospinal fluid (CSF). In the lab, this test takes only 5 minutes to 10 minutes to perform and helps to determine whether the meningitis is bacterial or viral. A final diagnosis is made by culturing the CSF or blood.[16,17]

TREATMENT

The treatment of meningitis should begin as soon as possible, and the drug of choice is penicillin, which is usually administered intravenously. Followup care is essential for household members or people such as respiratory therapists or medical personnel, who may have had direct contact with the patient's secretions or, who may have performed mouth-to-mouth resuscitation.

Infectious agent: Most common—Pneumococci, Haemophilus influenzae, Neisseria meningitidis, Staphylococcus aureus.
Mode of transmission: Direct contact with discharges from the nose or throat.
Incubation period: 2 days to 10 days.
Symptoms: Fever, headache, stiff neck, nausea and vomiting, rash.
Protective measures: Mask the patient or yourself.
Exposure followup: Necessary only if preventive measures were not followed, and you were involved in resuscitating, intubating, or suctioning the patient. Check with your medical director. If appropriate, Rifampin or Ampicillin may be prescribed.

Aseptic Meningitis

When symptoms are acute but no bacteria are present, the type of meningitis is aseptic or viral. Most cases of viral meningitis appear in patients under 40 years old and usually occur during the summer months. Transmission takes place through contact with infected feces, so that the risk of person-to-person contact is minimal.[20]

SIGNS AND SYMPTOMS

Signs and symptoms of aseptic meningitis include stiff neck and back, headache, fever, drowsiness, sore throat, and nausea. The patient may also complain of dizziness and abdominal or chest pains.[17]

DIAGNOSIS

Initially, diagnosis of aseptic meningitis is made based on symptoms and a gram stain. The gram stain will reveal a significant increase in white cells; no bacteria will be evident. Final diagnosis is made when the culture report is released.

TREATMENT

There is no specific drug therapy for aspectic or viral meningitis. This disease usually runs its course in a few days with no associated complications.

Infectious agent: Nonbacterial, virus strain.
Mode of transmission: Contact with infected feces.
Incubation period: Varies, depending on the strain of virus.
Symptoms: Fever, headache, stiff neck, nausea and vomiting, rash.
Protective measures: Since diagnosis is unknown, mask the patient or yourself.
Exposure followup: No followup is required.

■ MALARIA (JUNGLE FEVER)

Malaria is a sporozoan infection caused by protozoa of the genus *Plasmodium*, which includes the four species *P. vivax, P. malariae, P. knowlesi,* and *P. falciparum.*[21]

Malaria is transmitted by the bite of infected mosquitoes of the genus *Anopheles,* as well as through blood transfusions, transplacentally,[21] and through common needle use.[22]

In 1983, 803 cases of malaria were reported in the United States, which showed a slight decline compared to cases reported in 1982. Malaria may be brought to the United States by the following people: Refugees from endemic areas, military personnel assigned to endemic areas, and people who travel to endemic areas. Endemic areas for malarial illness include Africa, Asia, Central and South America, and the Caribbean islands.

Malarial patients with either acute or chronic illness usually present with symptoms of paroxysmal chills and high fever, headache, and sweating. The attacks of shivering and fever occur on a cyclic basis, every 48 hours to 72 hours, depending on the causative species. These symptoms are brought on by the release of merozoites into the blood when infested erythrocytes rupture. Figure 3-4 shows the malaria cycle. Infected patients may have an enlarged liver or spleen and may also show a "false positive" test for syphilis.[21]

Infectious agent: Sporozoan infection caused by several possible species of the genus *Plasmodium* (*P. vivax, P. falciparum, P. knowlesi,* and *P. malariae*).
Mode of transmission: Bite of a female *Anopheles* mosquito. Can be contracted by blood transfusion.
Incubation period: Weeks to months.
Symptoms: Periodic chills, fever, headache, sweating, enlarged spleen or liver.
Protective measures: Risks to EMS personnel who care for patients with a history of malaria are minimal. Even if you sustain a needle-stick injury, the chances of contracting the disease are very low.
Exposure followup: Document needle-stick injury only.

■ RABIES (HYDROPHOBIA)

Rabies is a disease caused by the rabies virus which, if acquired by humans, affects the central nervous system. Rabies can occur in any climate, is not seasonal, and occurs most often in wild animals such as bats, raccoons, skunks, and foxes. It can occur in domestic animals and, in this group, the cat is most often the source. Rabies is seen in animals, but rarely affects humans, with dog and cat bites remaining the main reasons for treating humans for exposure to rabies.

Rabies virus is excreted in saliva several days prior to full manifestation of the disease in an animal. The incubation period for this disease may be anywhere from 18 days to 1 year and is described as a slow-growing virus. The variance in the incubation period may be related to the location of the bite as well as to the amount of virus present in the saliva. A bite is not the only way to become exposed. Exposure may also occur as the result of virus coming in contact with mucous membranes or with the conjunctiva of the eye.

MALARIA (JUNGLE FEVER) ■ 33

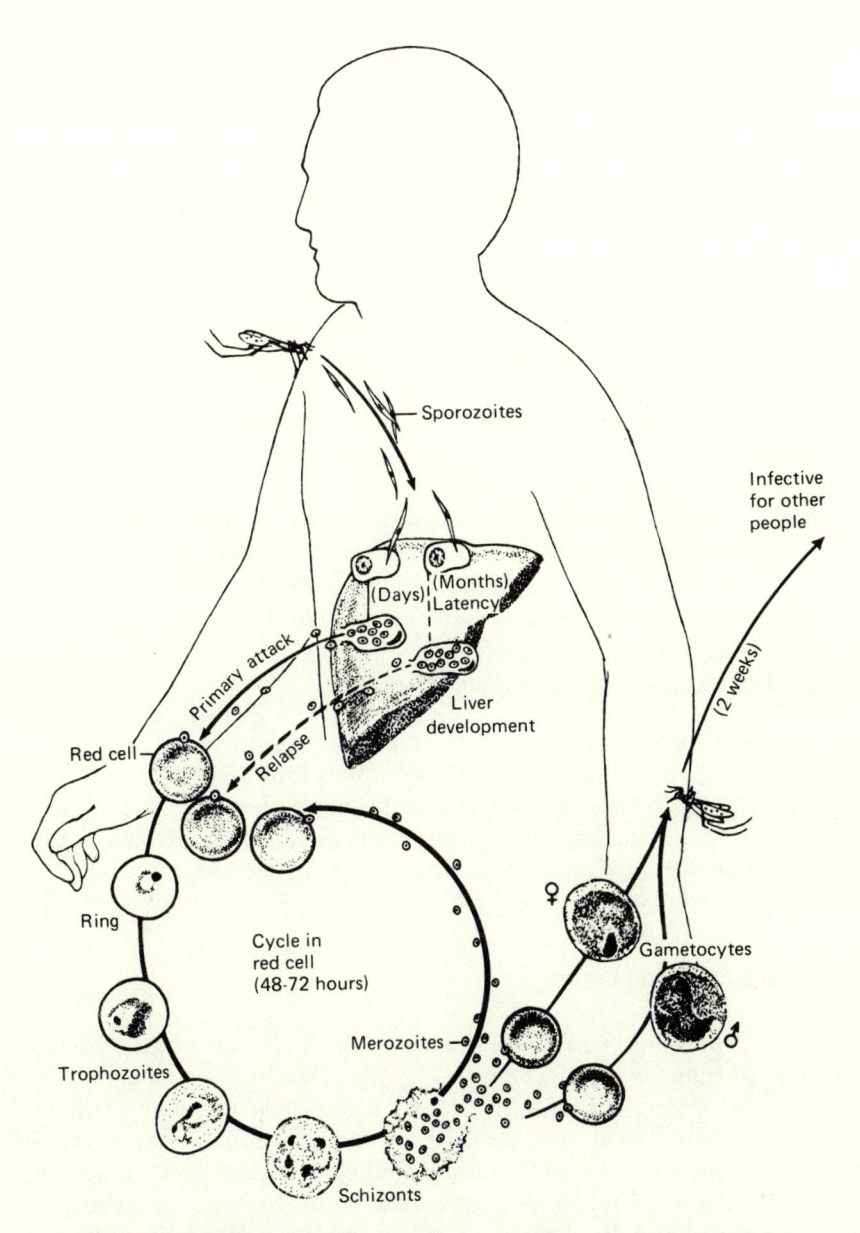

Figure 3-4. Malaria—the life cycle in man. (Miller LH: Transfusion malaria. In Greenwalt TJ, Jamieson CA (eds): Transmissible Diseases and Blood Transfusion. NY, Grune & Stratton, 1975)

Prophylaxis for rabies is based on the specific type of exposure, the animal species, and the circumstances that lead to the incident. Following a screening process to determine these factors, treatment is initiated.[23,24]

Infection agent: Rhabdovirus (rabies virus).
Mode of transmission: Direct contact with saliva of an infected animal. Virus may enter any area of broken skin, and may be transmitted by contact with the conjunctiva of an infected animal's eye. Human-to-human transmission has not been documented.
Incubation period: Usually 2 weeks to 8 weeks—may be longer. New information suggests that the virus grows slowly.
Symptoms: Headache, fever, malaise, neuromuscular irritability, convulsions; patient feels apprehensive.
Protective measures: Wear disposable gloves. Use good handwashing technique when in contact with saliva.
Exposure followup: Document exposure. Wash bite or scratches with soap and water. Tetanus prophylaxis should be given.[24]

Postexposure Immunization

Two types of immunizations are available: (1) Rabies immune globulin (RIG) and (2) human diploid cell rabies vaccine (HDCV). Both are considered safe and effective. Necessary immunization can be determined by type of exposure (see Table 3-2). The Public Health Department should be consulted.

■ SALMONELLA

Salmonella is an acute diarrhea illness that is characterized by a sudden onset of abdominal pain, diarrhea, nausea, vomiting, and fever. These symptoms may persist for several days. Diagnosis is made by examination of stool using culture technique. Salmonella can be excreted in stool for several weeks following illness, and some people can become chronic carriers.

Salmonella is found in wild as well as domestic animals. The pet turtle is a common source, but dogs and cats can also harbor the organism.

■ Table 3-2. POSTEXPOSURE TREATMENT FOR RABIES

The following recommendations are only a guide. In applying them, take into account the animal species involved, the circumstances of the bite or other exposure, the vaccination status of the animal, and presence of rabies in the region. Local or state public health officials should be consulted if questions arise about the need for rabies prophylaxis.

Animal Species	Condition of Animal at Time of Attack	Treatment of Exposed Person*
DOMESTIC Dog and cat	Healthy and available for 10 days of observation	None, unless animal develops rabies
	Rabid or suspected rabid	RIG and HDCV
	Unknown (escaped)	Consult public health officials. If treatment is indicated, give RIG and HDCV.
WILD Skunk, bat, fox, coyote, raccoon, bobcat, and other carnivores	Regard as rabid unless proven negative by laboratory tests.	RIG and HDCV
OTHER Livestock, rodents, and lagomorphs (rabbits and hares)	Consider individually. Local and state public health officials should be consulted on questions about the need for rabies prophylaxis. Bites of squirrels, hamsters, guinea pigs, gerbils, chipmunks, rats, mice, other rodents, rabbits, and hares almost never call for antirabies prophylaxis.	

*All bites and wounds should immediately be thoroughly cleansed with soap and water.
(Adapted from Rabies prevention. Epidemiology Bulletin, Sept. 1984)

This disease is transmitted by injection of the organism into contaminated food. Contamination usually involves foods that have been improperly prepared (i.e., undercooked chicken, raw sausage, or raw eggs).[23,25]

Infectious agent: Salmonella typhimurium (most common); 5 groups, 1500 serotypes.

Mode of transmission: Ingesting contaminated food or water; contact with infected feces.
Incubation period: 6 hours to 72 hours after ingesting contaminated food or water.
Symptoms: Nausea, vomiting, abdominal pain, and watery stool, which may contain blood or pus.
Protective measures: Wear disposable gloves. Use good handwashing technique when in contact with stools.
Exposure followup: Document exposure only if preventive measures were not used.

IMPETIGO

Impetigo is a superficial skin infection caused by either a staph or a strep infection. This infection follows three stages: First the lesions become vesicular (saclike); then they become pustular; finally they develop a crusted appearance. Lesions generally appear on the face and on the hands.[23,25]

This disease usually appears in young children in the summer and fall, and it occurs more often in hot temperature areas of the country than in cold temperature areas. It is transmitted by direct contact with an infected patient and, sometimes, by contact with contaminated objects (napkins, towels, plastic wading pools).

Impetigo is not associated with any complications.[25]

Infectious agent: Streptococcus (group B).
Method of transmission: Direct contact with lesions. Transmission by indirect contact with objects is rare, but sometimes occurs.
Incubation period: 1 day to 3 days.
Symptoms: Superficial skin infection—first appears as vesicles, then becomes pustular with crusts.
Protective measures: Wear disposable gloves and use good handwashing techniques.
Exposure followup: Document exposure. No treatment is recommended for exposure situations.

■ Childhood Diseases

■ MEASLES

The two types of measles viruses are rubeola, the red measles or 8-day measles, and rubella, the German measles or 3-day measles.

Rubeola (Red Measles)

Rubeola is a common childhood disease and is highly communicable. It is characterized by a fever, conjunctivitis, Koplik's spots (whitish gray spots on the buccal mucosa) and a dusky red, blotchy rash (Fig. 3-5). This rash usually appears on the face between the third day and seventh day and lasts about 4 days to 6 days. Rubeola is spread by direct contact with nasal or throat secretions; coughing or sneezing will create droplets in the air, which will contain the virus. Urine may also contain the virus. The incubation period is about 10 days, and the period during

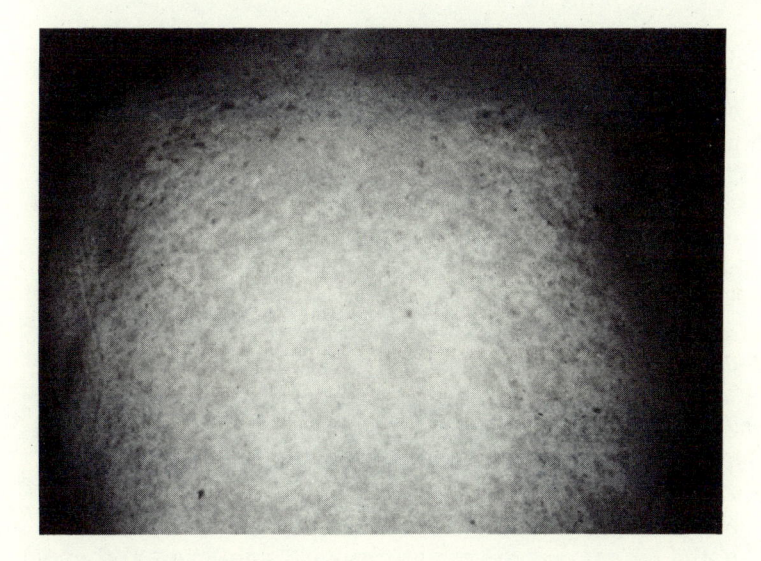

Figure 3-5. Rubeola.

which the individual is contagious is from the onset of the fever until 4 days after the rash appears. A person is immune to rubeola after vaccination or after contracting the disease. If documented exposure occurs, and if you are not immune, vaccination is recommended.

Infectious agent: Measles virus.
Mode of transmission: By droplets of direct contact with nasopharyangeal secretions or urine of an infected patient.
Incubation period: 8 days to 13 days.
Symptoms: Fever, conjunctivitis, dusky red, blotchy rash that usually starts on the face and spreads to the rest of the body, and Koplik's spots (whitish gray spots that are found on the buccal mucosa).
Protective measures: Wear disposable gloves and mask when in close contact with secretions of the mouth, nose, throat, and urine of an infected person.
Exposure followup: Document exposure. If you have never had the disease, you are not immune, therefore, vaccination is recommended.

Rubella (German Measles)

Rubella is a mild febrile disease characterized by a diffuse, macular rash (Fig. 3-6). This disease is spread by direct contact with nasopharyngeal secretions, and it incubates from 14 days to 21 days. Rubella is communicable from about 1 week before the rash appears until 4 days after it appears.

Rubella may be contracted by medical personnel who could then transmit the disease to others, which would be particularly dangerous to female personnel or family members. Pregnant personnel should be careful of exposing themselves to patients with rubella as contracting rubella in the first trimester may result in abnormal fetal development or congenital rubella syndrome. Vaccination is strongly recommended if a woman has never had rubella.

Diseases characterized by rash and fever are very difficult to diagnose. But remember, fever and rash are significant and may indicate an infectious process. The mode of transmission for

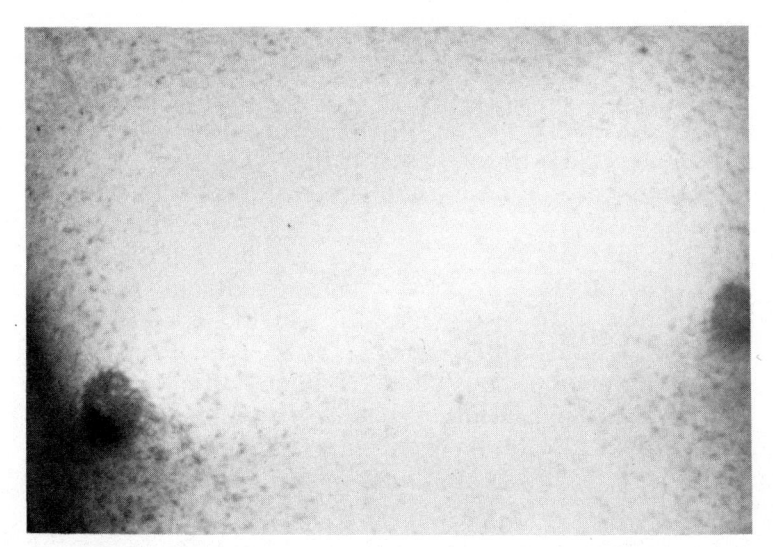

Figure 3-6. Rubella.

both measle viruses is through direct contact with nasopharyngeal secretions and droplets in the air, so protect yourself by wearing a mask. Also mask the patient whenever possible. Wear disposable gloves when directly contacting patient secretions. Good handwashing technique is also recommended.

Infectious agent: Rubella virus.
Mode of transmission: By droplets or direct contact with nasopharyngeal secretions, blood, urine, and stool of an infected person. Can be contracted by fetus from pregnant woman who has contracted the disease.
Incubation period: 14 days to 21 days.
Symptoms: Fever, diffuse and patchy rash, headache, conjunctivitis, swollen glands behind ears and base of skull.
Protective measures: Wear disposable gloves when handling secretions or excretions. Mask the patient or yourself.
Exposure followup: If preventive measures were not used, and you have not had the disease, document exposure and seek advice of your medical director.

■ MUMPS (INFECTIOUS PAROTITIS)

Mumps is characterized by fever and inflammation of the parotid glands, although other salivary glands may be involved. In approximately 30% of the cases, patients are asymptomatic. Mumps are most common in school age children, but can occur in nonimmune adults.

Complications of mumps are rare in children. However, about 20% of adult men who contract mumps will develop orchitis (inflammation of the testis). Orchitis usually affects only one testis and, although the question of sterility often arises following this complication, no clear documentation has been recorded.[26,27] One complication that has been documented is deafness, and in 10% of reported cases, meningoencephalitis (inflammation of the brain and meninges) has been a complication.

The incidence of mumps has greatly diminished since the vaccine was issued in 1967. The vaccine is routine in immunization programs and is usually given in conjunction with measles and rubella vaccines.[28]

Infectious agent: Mumps virus (myxovirus parotiditis).
Mode of transmission: Direct contact with saliva of an infected person.
Incubation period: 12 days to 26 days.
Symptoms: Fever, swelling and tenderness of the salivary glands. Inflammation of the testes in some adult males.
Protective measures: Disposable gloves when in contact with oral secretions. Good handwashing technique.
Exposure followup: Documentation of exposure if you have *not* had mumps. Seek advice of your medical director.[26]

■ CHICKENPOX (VARICELLA ZOSTER)

The causative agent for chickenpox is varicella, a member of the herpes virus family. This disease is usually spread from one child to another by contact with droplets in respiratory secretions. Nonimmune adults have acquired chickenpox from sick children, but cases have also been acquired from contact with individuals who have shingles (herpes zoster), a latent form of the same virus.

In children generally chickenpox is a mild disease that is characterized by a prodromal period (sore throat, low-grade fever, and headache) that lasts usually about 2 days. Then the rash appears, beginning on the face and back and spreading to the rest of the body. The rash then develops into vesicles, which will rupture and scab in the healing process. Chickenpox is communicable until the lesions are crusted and dried.

Although chickenpox is usually a mild disease in children, in adults complications are reported. Varicella pneumonia, for instance, has been reported as a complication, most often in men. This disease is especially severe if contracted by cancer patients.

Since chickenpox can be severe in adults even though basically it is a mild illness, and since varicella zoster immune globulin (VZIG) supplies are limited and costly, the decision to vaccinate an exposed person should be made on a case-by-case basis. Table 3-3 lists recommended criteria for making such decisions.

Infectious agent: Varicella zoster virus.
Mode of transmission: Droplets and airborne secretions from the respiratory tract.
Incubation period: 10 days to 21 days.
Symptoms: Fever, skin eruptions (vesicles) most often seen on areas of the body covered by clothing. (Fig. 3-7)
Protective measures: Wear disposable mask and gloves.

■ Table 3-3. EXPOSURE CRITERIA FOR ADMINISTERING VARICELLA ZOSTER IMMUNE GLOBULIN [29]

Types of Exposure to Infected Persons

Household contact (continuous)
Playmate contact (> 1 hour indoors).
Hospital contact (in two or four/bedroom) or prolonged face-to-face contact with an infectious staff member or patient
Newborn contact with mother who had onset of chickenpox 5 days or less before delivery or 48 hours after delivery
VZIG can be administered up to 96 hours after exposure, but preferable sooner.

42 ■ COMMUNICABLE DISEASES

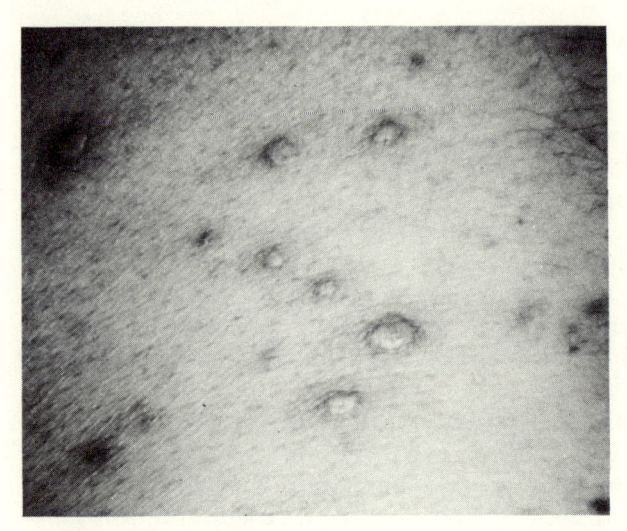

Figure 3-7. Chickenpox.

Exposure followup: Document exposure. If preventive measures have not been used, and if you have not had chickenpox, you may receive VZIG.[29]

■ PERTUSSIS (WHOOPING COUGH)

Pertussis (whooping cough) is usually seen in children under 7 years old. Disputing the belief that this disease no longer occurs in the United States, 2463 cases of pertussis were reported in 1983. Pertussis is a contagious respiratory disease and has a high mortality rate when contracted by children under 1 year of age.[30]

Small children probably contract pertussis from older children and young adults with decreased immunity levels who are ill and are the current source of illness to small children. This transmission may occur because booster shots are not given after 6 years of age. Without this stimulation from additional vaccine, immunity decreases.

Pertussis is caused by bacteria that affect the tracheabronchial tree and is characterized by an irritating cough. The cough gradually becomes paroxysmal (short, violent coughs with whoops) and may last for 1 month to 2 months. This cough is a "repeated" cough, and often the patient has difficulty catching a breath. When the coughing subsides, a high-pitched, inspiratory "whoop" sound is emitted, which may be followed by a clear, thick mucous. Causative bacteria reside in the nasopharyngeal secretions. The bronchioles, bronchi, trachea, and larynx become reddened, swollen, and covered by mucous.[31]

Outbreaks of pertussis are now occurring in the United States. These outbreaks stem from concern generated by studies conducted in Great Britain involving possible severe side-effects from the pertussis vaccine (DPT). In England, neurological complications in children who were vaccinated were characterized by seizures or prolonged screaming episodes that occurred within the first 24 hours after vaccination.[32,33] The media widely publicized these vaccine-related complications, and many alarmed parents requested that their children not be vaccinated.

The controversy over the pertussis vaccine made the medical community aware of several important factors: First, the studies that had been conducted in Britain needed to be reviewed; second, the studies conducted in the United States involving pertussis, as well as vaccines for other diseases, had shown that the incidence of neurologic complications was extremely low (less than 1:100,000).[32] Therefore, it was recommended that immunization with DPT should be continued. A vaccine shortage further complicates the situation, and immunization practices have been temporarily revised as follows:

1. All children under 12 months of age should be immunized.
2. Administration of boosters at 18 months and 4 years to 6 years of age should be postponed.
3. When an adequate supply of DPT becomes available, children will be recalled for imminizations.[34]

Infectious agent: Bordetella pertussis.
Mode of transmission: Contact with infected respiratory secretions.
Incubation period: 10 days to 16 days.
Symptoms: Nocturnal cough, a crowing whoop sound after deep inspiration, vomiting, infected conjunctivae, low-grade fever.

Protective measures: Wear a mask when in contact with secretions of mouth, nose, and throat.

Exposure followup: Document exposure. Contact medical director for recommended chemoprophylaxis. ISG or erythromycin may be indicated.

■ Sexually Transmitted Diseases

This section reviews the most common sexually transmitted diseases (STDs). STD is the new term for diseases that are transmitted by sexual contact. The change in terminology is an attempt to remove some of the social stigma associated with these diseases.

Gonorrhea and syphilis are the most common sexually transmitted diseases. However, other diseases, such as acquired immune deficiency syndrome (AIDS), cytomegalovirus disease (CMV), lice, scabies, hepatitis B, and herpes are also included in this category. Information on each of these diseases is included for review.

■ GONORRHEA

Gonorrhea may be the most widely studied STD in the past 20 years. In 1983 approximately one million cases of gonorrhea were reported in the United States, with the largest number of male cases appearing in men between the ages of 20 and 24 (homosexuality is a factor). In women the age group at highest risk appeared to be between 18 and 24 years of age.[35] In many STDs an increase in incidence has been related to the sexual revolution, the change in sexual values, and the use of intrauterine devices for contraception.

In men the primary symptoms are pain on urination and a urethral discharge. Complications associated with this disease are rare in males. In women symptoms may be absent. However, if present, they may include pain on urination, frequency of urination, lower abdominal pain, and discharge. In 40% of the cases reported in women, pelvic inflammatory disease has been the complication.

In the early stages of pregnancy gonococcal infection may cause sepsis in the fetus, resulting in rupture of the membranes and premature delivery. If infection is present at the time of delivery, the infant's eyes may be affected. Inflammation of the conjunctivae may occur 1 day to 7 days after delivery. This inflammation can be treated by instillation of silver nitrate solution or administration of erythromycin. A pregnant women with gonorrhea can be treated with penicillin G or amoxicillin to reduce infection in the fetus.[36] In recent years several strains of gonorrhea have been identified that are resistant to penicillin. In these cases treatment with spectinomycin is recommended.

Infectious agent: Neisseria gonorrhoeae.
Mode of transmission: Sexual contact, including oral–genital contact with an infected person.
Incubation period: 2 days to 7 days.
Symptoms: Urethral discharge, pain on urination (primary). Females may complain of lower abdominal pain.
Protective measures: When in contact with secretions of the genital tract, wear disposable gloves and use good handwashing technique.
Exposure followup: Document exposure. Followup treatment necessary only if preventive measures were not used. Contact your medical director.

■ SYPHILIS

Syphilis, an STD that plagued the people of ancient Egypt, was first distinguished from gonorrhea in the 18th century.[35] Syphilis is characterized by a primary lesion that appears about 3 weeks after exposure to the disease.

Syphilis occurs worldwide in young adults between 15 and 30 years of age. As with gonorrhea, the incidence of syphilis is greater in women than in men. This STD has also been increasing in incidence since the sexual revolution.[37]

Syphilis occurs in three stages: During the first, or primary, phase a lesion or chancre appears. The lesion is painless and can appear anywhere on the body. Even without treatment, this lesion will heal in 3 weeks to 6 weeks. The secondary stage begins 6 weeks to 8 weeks after the chancre appears. Lymph node enlargement may be noted, and a reddish brown rash may appear on the palms of the hands and soles of the feet. Mucous membranes may have gray white erosions. Additional symptoms include low-grade fever, headache, sore throat, and loss of appetite. The third, or latent, phase is the stage during which a blood serology test will be positive, but no other symptoms will be evident. Patients in the latent phase are generally not infectious.[38,39]

Treatment is divided into two approaches. One approach is treatment for primary, secondary, and latent syphilis of 1 year's duration. These people are given 2.4 million units of penicillin G in a single dose. The second treatment approach is for patients with syphilis of *more than* one year's duration. These patients are given 2.4 million units of penicillin once a week for 3 weeks.[40]

Infectious agent: A spirochete, *Treponema pallidum*.
Mode of transmission: Direct contact through sexual relations or blood of an infected person.
Incubation period: 3 weeks.
Symptoms: Initially, a painless lesion.
Protective measures: Wear disposable gloves and use a good handwashing technique when in contact with lesion or blood.
Exposure followup: Document exposure. Penicillin may be recommended depending on the type of exposure.[40]

■ AIDS (ACQUIRED IMMUNE DEFICIENCY SYNDROME)

Acquired immune deficiency syndrome (AIDS) is a disease that destroys the body's immune system. Normally the body's immune system protects us against infection and other diseases. When the immune system does not function properly, patients develop unusual infections.

AIDS was first recognized in 1978. However, since little time and money had been devoted to researching a disease affecting very few people at that time, information about AIDS was not available until 1981. Since then, due to the lobbying efforts of the Gay Alliance, significant amounts of money have been allocated for ongoing research. Consequently, the causative agent for AIDS has been identified as human T-cell lymphotropic virus type 3 (HIV*), a retrovirus.[41]

The news media have presented information about AIDS in a manner that has alarmed the general public. Some of this fear is not rooted in fact. For example, members of the general public are at small risk for contracting this disease. AIDS is primarily a sexually transmitted disease spread by bodily secretions (semen)[42] and through the blood. Homosexual and bisexual men—the primary group at risk—constitute 75% of AIDS cases. The second group at risk are street drug users, comprising 17% of AIDS cases.

Hemophiliacs, accounting for 1% of the cases, need factor VIII from plasma, which helps their blood to clot. In the past, blood donors who had AIDS passed the disease on to blood recipients, including hemophiliac patients. An additional 1% of AIDS cases are transfusion recipients.[42]

The remaining 6% of AIDS cases are comprised of women and children. Women may contract AIDS as a result of having sexual relations with infected bisexual men or, primarily, participation in IV drug use. AIDS has not developed in lesbian communities. New data have identified prostitutes as possible carriers of AIDS, and although male to female transmission is much more common, female to male transmission is presently being studied. One theory suggests that AIDS is linked primarily to homosexual men and the practice of rectal intercourse.

Some children have contracted AIDS. Many of these children were born to parents with histories of IV drug use, and 17 of the children reported had at least one Haitian parent. The remaining children had received blood transfusions.[42]

The symptoms of AIDS include a history of fever with profuse night sweats persisting for several months; fatigue and loss of appetitie persisting for more than 1 month; weight loss of 10 pounds to 20 pounds per month, not related to dieting; persistent diarrhea; presence of a herpes lesion for more than 1 month; persistent cough accompanied by shortness of breath; swollen lymph glands in the neck, axilla, and groin; and Kaposi's sarcoma—purplish colored bumps or lesions of various sizes appearing on the body.

The major age group at risk ranges between 22 years and 50

*HTLV-3 has been renamed HIV to give a consistent name to the virus.

years of age, with the mean age being 35 years old. AIDS is spreading to the general population, but is relatively confined to the high-risk groups. Although heterosexual transmission has occurred, it is uncommon, and it can be curtailed if the recommendations for safe sex are practiced. Recommendations for safe sex include:

1. Limit your number of sexual contacts.
2. Know your sexual partner and ask if he or she has a history of sexually transmitted diseases.
3. Men should use a condom.
4. Women should use a barrier method (diaphragm and a spermicidal foam or gel). The gel or foam should contain the chemical agent nonoxynol 9. This agent has been shown to kill hepatitis, herpes, and the HIV virus.[43]

The Centers for Disease Control (CDC) have published general guidelines for medical personnel to follow when caring for AIDS patients. These guidelines are reinforcements of currently recommended good practices and include the following:

1. Be cautious when handling needles and other sharp instruments.
2. Wear disposable gloves when handling body specimens, fluids, and secretions.
3. Blood spills should be treated promptly with a disinfectant solution of sodium hypochlorite (bleach).
4. Needles should be disposed of in a puncture-resistant container. Needles should not be cut or bent, as this creates an aerosol. Avoid recapping needles—this is when most sticks occur.
5. Wear cover gowns when exposed to an AIDS patient who is massively bleeding or who has bowel or bladder incontinence.
6. Use good handwashing technique.[44]

Some medical personnel have had direct exposure to AIDS patients. Sixty-five percent of these personnel had needle stick injuries, 16% had cuts from instruments, 14% had contact with mucosa, and 6% had contact with open lesions. The exposed personnel included nurses, physicians, phlebotomists, respiratory therapists, and laboratory and maintenance personnel. These personnel have been followed for over one year, and none has developed AIDS.

On December 14, 1984, Dr. Harold Jaffee of the Centers for Disease Control stated, "No case of AIDS in health care workers has been fully documented." He emphasized that the risk for health care workers still appeared to be "very, very small."[45,46]

The key to reducing cross infection of any of these diseases is to practice basic preventive measures—using good handwashing technique and wearing disposable gloves when in contact with blood and bodily secretions.

Infectious agent: A virus—human T-cell lymphotropic virus type 3 (HIV).
Mode of transmission: Contact with blood or bodily secretions, or sexual contact.
Incubation period: 2 months to 5 years.

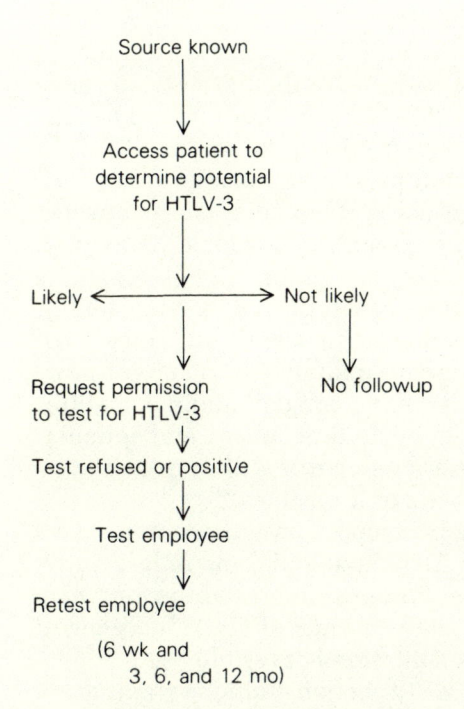

```
                    Source known
                         |
                         v
                 Access patient to
                 determine potential
                     for HTLV-3
                         |
                         v
   Likely <------------------------> Not likely
      |                                   |
      v                                   v
Request permission                   No followup
  to test for HTLV-3
      |
      v
Test refused or positive
      |
      v
  Test employee
      |
      v
 Retest employee
   (6 wk and
    3, 6, and 12 mo)
```

(Adapted from MMWR 34:681–695, November 15, 1985)

Symptoms: Fever with profuse night sweats, weight loss (10 lbs. to 20 lbs. per month), reddish purple skin lesions (Kaposi's sarcoma), pneumonia (caused by *pneumocystis carinii*).

Protective measures: Wear disposable gloves when in contact with blood or body fluids. Wash hands following patient care, even if gloves were used. Use portable CPR equipment (disposable airway and ambu bag), whenever possible. Purchasing "AIDS suits" or "AIDS kits" is not recommended and is an additional expense. Wear disposable gowns only when clothing may be soiled with blood or body fluids.[44]

Exposure followup: Should you sustain a contaminated needle stick, report this to your medical director. The recommended followup, depending on the type of exposure, may involve HTLV-3 antibody testing following the exposure and at intervals of 3 months, 6 months, and 12 months.

■ CYTOMEGALOVIRUS INFECTION

Cytomegalovirus (CMV), a member of the herpes virus family, is a frequent cause of infection in both children and adults. This infection is usually contracted during the perinatal period following congenital infection. In most cases, people with CMV are asymptomatic.[47] In the United States and western Europe, 30% to 80% of the population have antibodies for CMV, which indicates previous infection.[48]

Primary or initial infection may be followed by persistent or intermittent excretion of virus, which is significant since most patients are asymptomatic.[49] Approximately 5% to 10% of newborns with CMV infections also have congenital abnormalities such as deafness, mental deficiency, hydrocephaly, and epilepsy. An additional 10% to 20% of these newborns will develop abnormalities within the first few years of their lives.[50]

CMV infections may also be seen in immunocompromised patients, such as patients with AIDS, leukemia, and renal failure, as well as transplant patients. Post-transfusion infections may also occur in CMV patients. The presence of CMV in venereal cultures suggests that anal transmission is possible.

Generally symptoms of CMV infections mimic symptoms of mononucleosis.[49] Serious risks for medical personnel are unsupported by data.

Infectious agent: Cytomegalovirus, a herpes virus.
Mode of transmission: Direct contact with secretions from cervix, semen, blood, feces, saliva, and urine.
Incubation period:

>Perinatal infection—4 weeks to 12 weeks
>Post-transfusion infection—3 weeks to 8 weeks
>Sexual infection—4 weeks to 8 weeks

Symptoms: Fever, swollen lymph glands, rash, sore throat, liver and spleen enlargement.
Preventive measures: Wear disposable gloves. Use good hand-washing technique when in contact with secretions.
Exposure followup: Document exposure. Increased risk to medical personnel is unsupported.

■ LICE (PEDICULOSIS)

Lice are divided into three types, according to the areas of the body they inhabit:

Pediculus humanus capitis—the head louse
Pediculus humanus corporis—the body, or clothes, louse
Phthirus pubis—the pubic, or crab, louse[51]

These parasitic lice have six legs and reproduce by laying eggs. Head and pubic lice attach their eggs to hair shafts on the human body with a cementlike substance. The body louse attaches its eggs to the clothing of a person and then feeds off the person.

In order to survive, lice require a blood meal every 24 hours to 48 hours, although they may live without a human host for 2 days or more.

Infectious agents: Pediculus humanus capitis (head louse), *Phthirus pubis* (crab louse), *Pediculus humanus corporis* (body louse).
Mode of transmission:

>*Head & body louse*—close contact with infested persons or their personal items, such as scarves, hats, combs, and furniture.
>*Crab louse*—sexual contact, bedding, or clothing (rarely by toilet seat).

Incubation period: 1 week to 2 weeks.
Symptoms: Itching; nits (eggs) may be seen with the naked eye.
Protective measures: Wear disposable gloves when possible.
Exposure followup: Document exposure. Clothing should be washed in hot water. Wear gloves and gown when cleaning patient contact areas following the transport. Use Kwell lotion as directed, or over-the-counter medications as directed.[52]

■ SCABIES

The scabies mite has eight legs. The male usually lives on the surface of the skin, while the female burrows under the skin to lay her eggs. Scabies is difficult to diagnose because infested patients are often asymptomatic for up to 4 weeks. Irritation develops as a result of the mites' waste products deposited under the skin. Diagnosis is made by skin scrapings or skin biopsy, which will reveal mites.[53,54]

Infectious agent: Sarcoptes scabiei, a small mite.
Mode of transmission: Skin to skin contact. Extensive hands-on contact is usually required for transmission to occur.
Incubation period: 2 weeks to 6 weeks
Symptoms: Inflammation and itching (worse at night)—usually located on breasts, abdomen, elbows, ankles, lower buttocks, external genitalia, and occasionally between the fingers.
Protective measures: Wear disposable gloves when possible. Use thorough handwashing technique.
Exposure followup: Document exposure. Use Kwell lotion as directed by physician.[54] Some over-the-counter medications are available (R&C Lotion, RID).

■ Herpes Viruses

Herpes is a small virus that contains deoxyribonucleic acid (DNA). Members of the herpes virus family include: herpes simplex (types 1 and 2), herpes zoster, cytomegalovirus, varicella (chickenpox), and the Epstein–Barr virus, which causes mononucleosis.[55] This section discusses herpes simplex (types 1 and 2) and herpes zoster.

■ HERPES SIMPLEX (TYPES 1 AND 2)

Herpes viruses usually enter the body through mucous membranes (lips or genital areas) or breaks in the skin. Once inside the body, a herpes virus attaches itself to the surface of a host cell. Then it penetrates the cell wall and multiplies until it is released outside the cell. Once outside the cell, the body's immune system activates and responds. Some herpes virus retreats into the nerve fiber and escapes detection. The virus particles then travel down the nerve and inhabit the base of the nerve's ganglia where the virus remains dormant, sometimes indefinitely, protected by nerve tissue.

Infection with herpes virus becomes evident when lesions appear. These lesions are triggered apparently by emotional or physical stress, sunlight, or in conjunction with a viral illness.

Usually 2 days to 3 days before a lesion appears the patient will experience a localized itching, tingling, and burning sensation. This prelesion phenomenon is called *prodrome*[56] and is a signal that the virus is being shed in a small amount. A patient is communicable from the time the virus begins shedding until the lesion is completely crusted and dry.

Before 1960 it was thought that type 1 lesions included any lesions that appeared above the waist, and type 2 lesions included those that appeared below the waist. However, recent information indicates that through participation in oral sex, either type of herpes lesions can appear at either location of the body, making it difficult to differentiate between type 1 and type 2. Nevertheless, 80% of herpes simplex viral infections that occur above the waist are type 1 infections, and 20% are type 2 infections. Whether a specific lesion is type 1 or type 2 must be determined in the laboratory with the aid of an electron microscope.

How do the lesions evolve? First, a small patch of erythema (redness) appears and develops into a thin-walled vesicle filled with clear fluid. Usually several vesicles are grouped together and are preceded by a prodrome (warning signal).[57]

54 ■ COMMUNICABLE DISEASES

Approximately 80% of the population have been exposed to herpes. Some people develop lesions, and some do not. Although asymptomatic carriers do not develop lesions, they still shed virus in their oral secretions or genital tracts. Therefore, medical personnel may contract herpes from asymptomatic patients as well as patients with obvious lesions.

Oral Herpes

Herpes lesions that appear on or around the mouth are often called "cold sores" or "fever blisters." When lesions appear in this area, the trigeminal nerve is affected by the virus. Figure 3-8 demonstrates an oral herpes lesion.

Infectious agent: Herpes simplex virus, type 1 (can be type 2, depending on exposure).
Mode of transmission: Direct contact with lesions or with oral mucous membranes.
Incubation period: 2 days to 12 days—may vary individually.

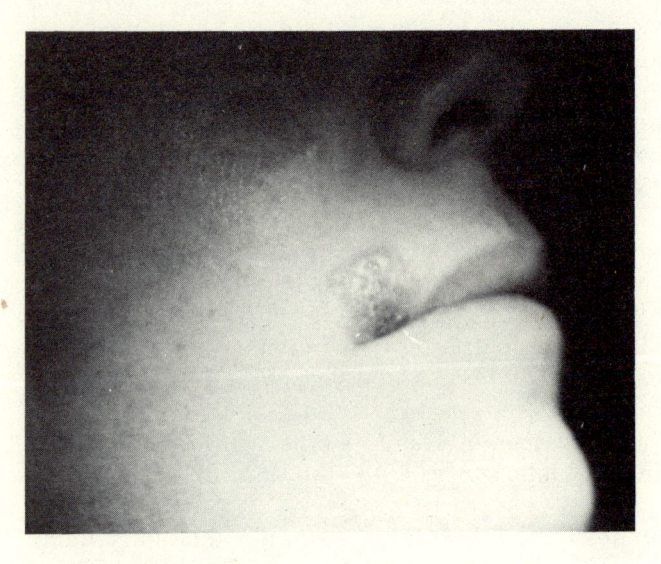

Figure 3-8. Oral herpes.

Symptoms: Itching, tingling at site, followed by appearance of a lesion and low-grade fever.
Protective measures: Wear disposable gloves when in contact with a lesion or mucous membranes. Use good handwashing technique.
Exposure followup: None. Document exposure.

Herpetic Whitlow

In Figure 3-9 note that the tip of the finger is red and swollen with a white patchy area in the center. This is called herpetic whitlow, a recently recognized herpes infection of the finger. Herpetic whitlow is characterized by pain and swelling, but otherwise behaves as other herpes viruses behave. Herpetic whitlow also will appear and disappear and, at present, is incurable. An individual who develops herpetic whitlow may be unable to work for at least 1 week with each recurrence.

Breaks in the skin may provide an entry point for the virus from oral secretions of infected patients. Therefore, medical personnel who have torn cuticles, paper cuts, or puncture wounds

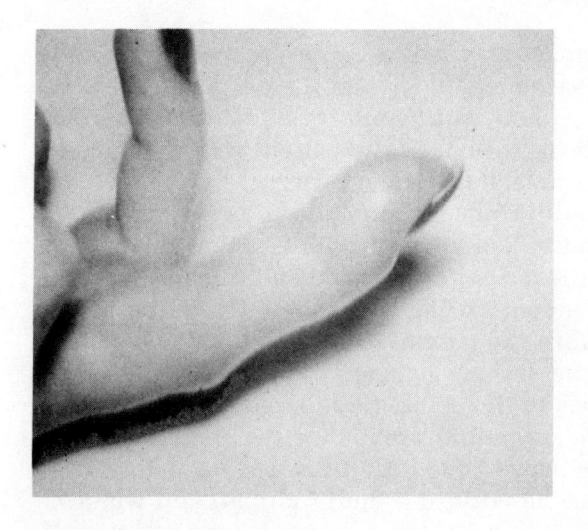

Figure 3-9. Herpetic whitlow.

on their fingers should wear disposable gloves when involved with the following procedures: Passing an airway, putting in an esophageal obturator airway (EOA), clearing an airway, or suctioning a patient.

Protective and preventive measures should include wearing disposable gloves whenever possible and using a good handwashing technique.[58]

Infectious agent: Herpes simplex virus, type 1.
Mode of transmission: Virus enters through breaks in the skin after contact with oral or tracheal secretions of patient shedding herpes virus.
Incubation period: 2 days to 12 days—may vary individually.
Symptoms: Redness, swelling, tenderness, nerve impairment of the finger or hand.
Protective measures: Wear disposable gloves on both hands when in contact with oral or treacheal secretions. Use good handwashing technique.[58]
Exposure followup: Document exposure. As with other herpes virus infections, only symptomatic treatment is available.

Genital Herpes (Male)

Figure 3-10 demonstrates genital herpes in a male. Note the deep ulcerated areas along the penis. If you were doing an assessment on this patient, you would first ask him if he had pain associated with the lesions. If the patient was having pain, herpes would be probable. If the patient was not having pain, his lesions could be syphilitic chancres.

When is this individual communicable? From the time of the prodrome until the lesions are crusted and dried. Advise the patient to wear a condom during sexual relations if he is in a prodromal phase. Warn the patient to abstain from sexual relations once the active lesions appear.[56] Many herpes experts believe that the pores in the condom are large enough to allow entry of the virus and, therefore, are ineffective in protecting the partner. Basically, however, the only time a male with genital herpes is communicable is during the prodrome and when he has active lesions.

The sacral nerve is affected by the genital herpes virus. The

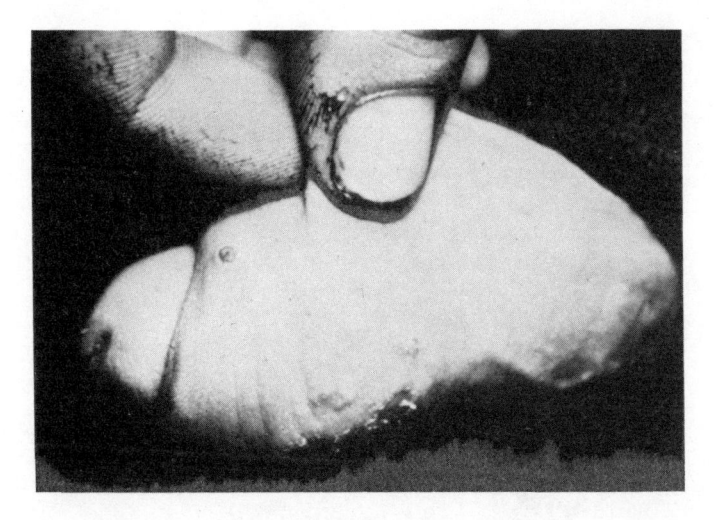

Figure 3-10. Genital herpes—male.

initial outbreak of this virus lasts approximately 21 days. Eighty percent of genital lesions are caused by type 2 virus; 20% of genital lesions are type 1 infections.

Genital Herpes (Female)

Figure 3-11 demonstrates genital herpes in the female and reveals a deep ulcerated area with some pustules. If you are ever involved in a field delivery, and you note any lesions such as these, communicate that information to the dispatcher so that the hospital can be notified to take the proper precautions. In this situation, as the baby passes through the birth canal, he or she is exposed to drainage from the lesions and may develop herpes. The mortality rate for such infants has been about 96%. However, a new drug, acyclovir, has helped reduce the mortality rate to approximately 73%. In the United States the incidence of herpes in newborns is small (2%), but is still devastating for the infant. Infants are more susceptible to herpes because their immune systems are not fully developed. If death is not incurred, blindness or severe neurological damage may result. Many infants develop recurring localized lesions.

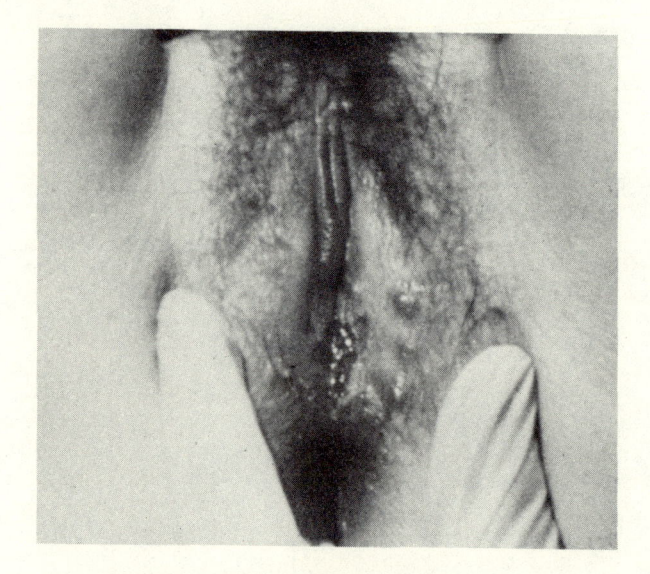

Figure 3-11. Genital herpes—female.

If a woman has a history of herpes, the decision to perform a cesarean section depends on certain criteria. If she has active lesions at the time of delivery, a c-section should be performed to prevent the baby from being exposed to the virus in the birth canal. However, if the woman's membranes have been ruptured for 8 hours or more, she may deliver her baby vaginally, assuming that the virus has ascended into the uterine cavity.[59] If the patient has a history of herpes and there are no active lesions at the time of delivery, she may have a normal vaginal delivery with no risk to the infant. Many people have the misconception that once a woman with genital herpes has had a c-section she will always have to have a c-section; this is not always true.

Infectious agent: Herpes simplex virus, type 2 (can be type 1, depending on the exposure).
Mode of transmission: Sexual contact with lesions or skin to lesion contact. Virus enters through breaks in the skin. This virus is not airborne and can not be contracted from toilet seats, pools, hot tubs, or sheets.
Incubation period: 2 days to 12 days—may vary individually.
Symptoms: Burning, itching, tingling, tenderness at the site,

dysuria, fever, swollen glands, thin white discharge, lesions that become ulcerated on penis, vulva, buttocks, thighs.

Protective measures: Wear disposable gloves when in contact with lesions. Use good handwashing technique.

Exposure followup: None. Document exposure. If herpes is contracted, only symptomatic treatment is available.

MANAGEMENT OF HERPES SIMPLEX

Because herpes is incurable, people with genital lesions will have recurring outbreaks. Consequently, many of these people are emotionally devastated. Support groups have been established throughout the United States to help herpes patients deal with the disease's emotional aspects. Although herpes is not fatal, it is inconvenient and necessitates a change in lifestyle. To change the stigma surrounding herpes, the facts should be learned and the myths disputed.

Transferring herpes virus from one part of the body to another is called *autoinfection*. Although rare, autoinfection is possible usually only during primary infection. During recurrence the body's immune system eliminates virus particles that could be transferred. If you have an outbreak of herpes and want to reduce the possibilities for autoinfection, avoid contact with lesions and practice good handwashing technique.

Although there is no cure for herpes, a recently available antiviral agent, acyclovir (Zovirax), helps reduce the discomfort of symptoms and aids the healing process.

Studies indicate that, as a topical ointment, acyclovir is effective in reducing pain and viral shedding as well as in aiding the healing time for initial herpes infections. In intravenous form, acyclovir is used in the treatment of newborns and immunocompromised patients with severe herpes infections.[60] Oral acyclovir is now available in capsule form. Studies have shown that when taken daily for a prescribed period of time these capsules will prevent recurrences, offering the greatest hope yet for herpes patients. However, for recurring lesions, the best treatment is to keep the affected area clean and dry.

A herpes vaccine may be available within 3 years to 5 years, but it would not benefit patients currently infected with herpes.[61]

■ HERPES ZOSTER

Figure 3-12 illustrates shingles, a member of the herpes family known as herpes zoster. Note how this virus develops on a single nerve pathway. As previously stated, herpes viruses are elusive, often remaining dormant for long periods. Shingles differ from other herpes infections in that the lesions contain live chickenpox virus. In some people, the virus from childhood chickenpox remains dormant on the dorsal nerve and years later, during chronic illness or physical stress, an outbreak of shingles may occur.[57]

As with other herpes lesions, shingles are painful. An outbreak may last as long as 2 weeks to 3 weeks and can recur. Outbreaks of shingles are common in immunocompromised patients and nursing home patients.

Medical personnel who have not had chickenpox could contract chickenpox while transporting a patient with shingles. A person can not contract shingles from patients who have shingles—chickenpox is the risk. In this situation, it is essential to

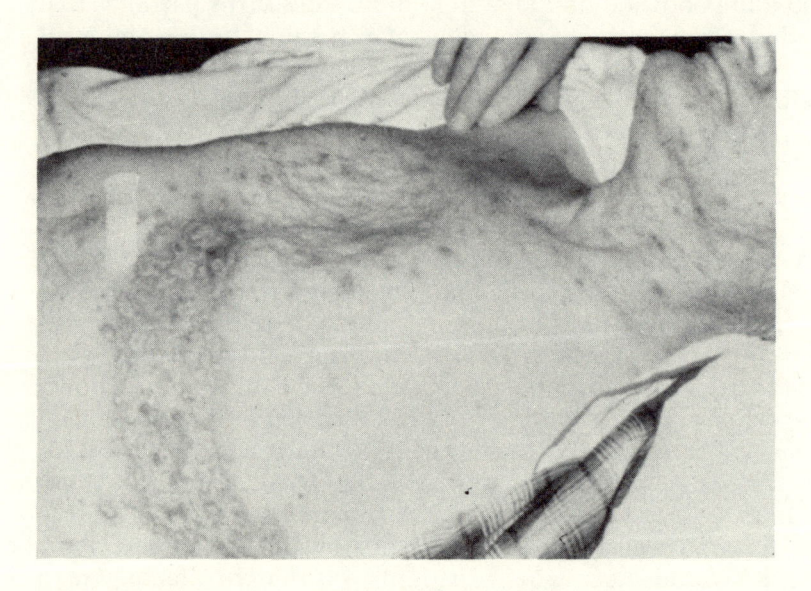

Figure 3-12. Herpes zoster (shingles).

wear disposable gloves and use good handwashing techniques, especially if you must have contact with the lesions.

Normally chickenpox is transmitted via respiratory secretions. However, with shingles the virus is transmitted only through direct contact.

Infectious agent: Varicella zoster (chickenpox virus).
Mode of transmission: Direct contact with infected vesicles.
Incubation period: 2 weeks to 3 weeks. If you are not immune, you could develop chickenpox.
Symptoms: Unilateral rash with eruptions, burning pain, and itching.
Protective measures: Wear disposable gloves when in contact with draining lesions. Use good handwashing technique.
Exposure followup: Document exposure. Zoster immune globulin (ZIG) may prevent or modify disease, but is recommended in few cases.

■ References

1. Riley RL: The hazard is relative: Editorial: Am Rev Respir Dis 96:623, 1967
2. Farer LS: Incidence and epidemiology of tuberculosis in the 1980s: Guidelines for the diagnosis of tuberculosis infection. Symposium proceedings, pp 7–14. New York, Parke-Davis, Div. Warner-Lambert, Nov 1983
3. Atuk NO, Hart AD, Hart EW: Close monitoring is essential during isoniazid prophylaxis. South Med J 70:156–159, 1977
4. Reichman LB: Roundtable discussion. Symposium on Worldwide Incidence of Tuberculosis, New York, Parke-Davis, Div. Warner-Lambert, 1983
5. Daniel TM, Mahmoud AAF, Warren KS: Algorithms in the diagnosis of and management of exotic diseases, XVI: Tuberculosis. J Infec Dis 134:417–421, 1976
6. Farer LS: Tuberculosis: What the physician should know. American Lung Association, 1982
7. Suboptional response to hepatitis B vaccine given by injection into the buttocks. MMWR 34:105–108, 1985
8. West KH: The dilemma—hepatitis B: What is it all about? JORRI 2:8–12, 1982
9. Centers for Disease Control: Hepatitis Surveillance Report No. 48, 1982

10. Dienstag JL, Ryan DM: Occupational exposure to hepatitis b virus in hospital personnel: Infection or immunization? Am J Epidemiol 115:26-39, 1982
11. Craven DE et al: Hepatitis B expsoure in emergency medical personnel. Am J Med 75:269-272, 1983
12. Tabor E, Ponzetto A, et al: Does delta agent contribute to fulminent hepatitis? Lancet, 765, April 1983
13. Redeker AG: Delta agent and Hepatitis B. Ann Intern Med 98:542-543, 1983
14. Immune globulins for protection against viral hepatitis. MMWR 30:423-428, 1981
15. Post exposure prophylaxis of hepatitis B. MMWR 30:285-289, 1984
16. Axnich K, Yarbrough M: Infection Control: An Integrated Approach, pp 493-539. St. Louis, CV Mosby, 1984
17. Hoeprich PD: Infectious Diseases, 2nd ed, pp 889-901. Hagerstown, Harper & Row, 1977
18. Bell NE, Selber DL: Meningococcal meningitis: Past and present concepts. Milit Med 136:601, 1971
19. Goldschneider I et al: Human immunity to the meningococcus. J Exp Med 129:1307, 1966
20. Garner JS, Simmons BP: CDC guidelines for isolation precautions in hospitals. Infect Control 4:308, 1983
21. US Department of Health and Human Services: Malaria Surveillance. Annual Summary, 1984
22. Hoeprich PD: Infectious diseases, 2nd ed, pp 1075-1087. Hagerstown, Harper & Row, 1977
23. Benenson AS: Control of Communicable Diseases in Man. Washington, DC, American Public Health Association, 1975
24. Immunization Practices Advisory Committee: Rabies. MMWR, 33(28), July 1984
25. Weherle PF, Top FH: Communicable Diseases and Infectious Diseases. St. Louis, CV Mosby, 1982
26. Krugman S, Katz, SL: Infectious Diseases of Children, 7th ed, pp 195-199. St. Louis, CV Mosby, 1981
27. Werner, CA: Mumps orchitis and testicular atrophy. Ann Intern Med 32:1066-1074, 1950
28. Koplan JP, Preblud SR: A benefit-cost analysis of mumps vaccine. Am J Dis Child 136:362-364, 1982
29. Varicella-zoster immune globulin for the prevention of chickenpox. Epidemiology Bulletin 84(3):1-6, 1984
30. Nelson JD: The changing epidemology of pertussis in young infants. Am J Dis Child 132:371-373, 1978
31. Miller FN: Pathology, p 109. Boston, Little, Brown & Co, 1978

REFERENCES ■ 63

32. Fenichel GM: Editorial: The pertussis vaccine controversy. Arch Neurol, 40:193-194, 1983
33. The pertussis vaccine. Am Fam Physician 27:127-128, 1983
34. Diphtheria-tetanus-pertussis vaccine shortage. MMWR, 33:695-696, 1984
35. Hook EW, Holmes KK: Gonococcal infection. Ann Intern Med, 102:229-243, 1985
36. Treatment of sexually transmitted diseases. Med Lett, 26:5-100, 1984
37. Benenson AS: Control of communicable diseases in man, 12th ed, pp 314-317. Washington, DC, American Public Health Association, 1975
38. Hoeprich PD: Infectious Diseases, 2nd ed, pp 517-535. Hagerstown, Harper & Row, 1977
39. Mandell GL, Douglas RG, Bennett JE: Principles and Practice of Infectious Diseases, pp 151-153. New York, John Wiley & Sons, 1979
40. Sexually transmitted diseases treatment guidelines. MMWR 31:Supplement No. 25, 33s-60s, 1982
41. Commentary: The acquired immunodeficency syndrome. JAMA, 252(15):2037-2043, 1984
42. Update: Acquired immunodeficiency syndrome (AIDS). MMWR, 33(24):337-339, June 22, 1984
43. Heterosexual transmission of human t-lymphotropic virus type-111/lymphadenopathy-associated virus. MMWR, September 20, 34:37:561-562, 1985
44. Acquired immune deficiency syndrome (AIDS) precautions for clinical and laboratory staffs. MMWR, 31(43):577-579, 1982
45. Health care workers exposed via paunteral or mucous-membrane routes to blood and body fluids of patients with AIDS. MMWR 33(13):181-182, April 6, 1984
46. Valenti, WM: Update on AIDS. Infection Control, 6(2):85-86, 1985
47. Benenson AS: Control of Communicable Diseases in Man, pp 99-102. Washington, DC, American Public Health Association, 1975
48. Lang DJ: Cytomegalovirus immunization: Status, prospects, and problems. Rev Infect Dis, 2:449-458, 1980
49. Hoeprich PD: Infectious Diseases, pp 628-632. Hagerstown, Harper & Row, 1977
50. Stagno S et al: Maternal cytomegalo-virus infection and perinatal transmission. Clin Obstet Gyn, 25:568-576, 1982
51. Miller FN: Pathology, p. 219. Boston, Little, Brown & Co, 1978
52. Minster J: Nursing management of patients with scabies and lice. Nurs Clin North Am, 15:747-756, 1980

53. Chapel TA: Scabies and pediculosis: Hospitalized mites and lice. Asepsis, 6(1):13–21, 1984
54. Marianette MK, Spitz S: Communicable disease protocols for the emergency department and employee health service: A cooperative venture of APIC–Rochester Finger Lakes Educational Comm. AJIC, 10(4):43A–45A, November 1982
55. Rapp F: Herpes viruses, venereal disease, and cancer. SCORE, 5:14–18, 1980
56. Waimboodt L: Herpes, the shock, the stigma, the ways you can ease the emotional pain. RN, May:47–49, 1983
57. Hoeprich PD: Infectious Diseases, pp 726–743. Hagerstown, Harper & Row, 1982
58. West KH: Herpetic whitlow: A new concern for health care professionals. JORRI, April, Vol 3:6–8, 1983
59. Whitley RJ et al: The natural history of herpes simplex virus infection of mother and newborn. Pediatrics, 66:489–494, 1980
60. Macek C: IV and oral acyclovir surpass topical use. JAMA, 248:2942–2948, 1982
61. Parks WP, Rapp F: Prospects for herpes vaccination: Safety and efficacy considerations. Prog Med Vis, 21:188–206, 1975

Caring for Your Rescue Vehicle, Supplies, and Equipment 4

■ RECOMMENDATIONS FOR CLEANING YOUR RESCUE VEHICLE

Your vehicle may be a source of infection, because bacteria can reside on equipment surfaces. When you clean your vehicle routinely, you help reduce the possibility of contacting and transferring these bacteria.

Cleaning your vehicle involves two important steps—washing and disinfecting. Cleaning is defined as the physical removal of visible surface debris. The use of soap and water and the application of elbow grease is essential, because disinfection can not be accomplished unless surface debris has been removed. After washing your vehicle, disinfect the internal surfaces with chemicals to kill infectious pathogens and reduce the possibility of cross contamination.

The approach to this procedure should be a common sense approach. Clean the floor and walls on a regular basis or when heavily soiled. You do not have to disinfect the walls and floors, since probably your patients will not be in direct contact with these parts of the vehicle. You do need to pay special attention to washing and disinfecting actual work areas, however, since such areas include surfaces you may touch while treating patients. Bacteria and viruses from these surfaces could be transferred to the patient.

Although no specific disinfectant solutions are recommended, the Centers for Disease Control (CDC) suggests using an Environmental Protection Agency (EPA) registered germicidal/viricidal agent. Table 4-1 reviews the most common solutions available. A key factor in selecting a solution is its effect on

Table 4-1. GUIDE TO USING DISINFECTANTS

Helpful hints:

1. If you are using a detergent or disinfectant compound solution, clean the item before disinfection to remove blood, tissue, or secretions.
2. Make a fresh solution whenever possible, following manufacturer's instructions. Mark date and time prepared and the date the solution will expire.
3. Always store solutions according to the manufacturer's guidelines.

Agents	Purpose	Considerations
Isopropyl alcohol (70%–90%)	Bactericidal Effective against staph, strep, and TB. Ineffective against spores.	Avoid skin irration, wear gloves. Don't immerse rubber or plastic articles. Because alcohol evaporates quickly, use disinfected object immediately. Agent loses effectiveness when evaporated.
Chlorine	Bactericidal Effective against *Salmonella*, TB, hepatitis virus, *Staph aureus*, and strep. Used for patient-care equipment, such as bedpans, urinals, and thermometers, as well as for special general housekeeping chores. Also used in dialysis areas.	To avoid skin irritation, wear gloves when using. Do not use on items having close contact with patient's mucous membranes. Avoid using on metal articles to prevent discoloration and corrosion in some cases. Prepare fresh solution each time and use it immediately. Discard what remains.
Glutaraldehyde	Bactericidal Effective against staph and strep, TB, viruses, and bacterial spores. Used to disinfect respiratory therapy equipment, lensed instruments, polythylene tubing, and dialysis equipment.	To avoid skin irritation, wear gloves when using. Store in a cool place. Use in a well-ventilated room. Activate before using. When activated, agent changes color. Read manufacturer's instructions carefully.

■ Table 4-1. GUIDE TO USING DISINFECTANTS (Continued)

Agents	Purpose	Considerations
Phenol	Bactericidal Effective against staph, strep and *Salmonella* organisms, some viruses, and TB. Less effective against spores. Used for patient-care equipment, such as bedpans and urinals, aswell as for general housekeeping.	Immerse article in agent (2% alkaline) for about 10 hours to ensure effectiveness against bacterial spores. To avoid skin irritation, wear gloves when using. Do not use on articles that have close contact with the patient's mucous membranes. Reactivates when exposed to moisture
Quats (Quaternary ammonium compounds)	Bactericidal Effective against staph and strep. Less effective against *Salmonella* organisms, and ineffective against TB and spores. Used for patient-care equipment, such as bedpans and urinals, as well as for general housekeeping.	Avoid using with soap. Soap reduces agent's effectiveness. Do not use for antisepsis. Pour directly on item to be cleaned. Cleaning clothes will absorb agent.

equipment surfaces. For example, chlorine is inexpensive but will cause clouding on Plexiglas and corrosion of metal with prolonged use. Always review literature from the company that manufactures the product. If there is not a complete list of organisms that the product should kill included with the product, request additional information from the manufacturer.[1,2]

If possible, coordinate your cleaning supplies with the hospital that your system services. Two possible advantages of such an arrangement are using their solutions or purchasing solutions through the hospital to save money. The personnel in central supply, purchasing, and infection control can probably advise you regarding purchasing products that will meet your needs.

Communicable Disease Transports

After transporting a patient either suspected of or diagnosed as having a communicable disease, clean and disinfect your vehicle. If you clean your vehicle after each transport, however, you will reduce the necessity for extensive followup of cleaning and disinfecting. As previously discussed, only wipe down high-contact areas, which should require about 5 minutes to 10 minutes. Vehicles do not need to be aired. According to the CDC, "airing is not an effective terminal disinfectant procedure and is not necessary."[1]

Items that were in contact with infectious material require special handling or bagging. For example, if your patient had measles, items that had been in contact with respiratory secretions would be considered contaminated.

Out of service or down time should be minimal. In most cases, you can quickly clean after delivering your patient to the emergency department or while enroute to your next call.[2]

CLEANING AND AIRING

Strip all linen and bag according to area hospital protocol. Clean all high-contact areas with a germicidal agent. Airing your vehicle is unnecessary.

BAGGING PROCEDURES

All items that have been in direct contact with respiratory secretions, oral secretions, or wound drainage should be considered infectious and, therefore, require special care. The procedure for bagging these items is as follows:

1. Wear disposable gloves.
2. Place all dressings or tissues in a bag and mark them for incineration.
3. Linen should be placed in either a water-soluble bag or a linen bag. Then this bag should be placed into a plastic or linen bag marked *isolation*.

Bagging procedures may vary in each hospital. Be aware of the system used in your service area and be sure that bags are available on your unit or in the emergency department for easy access. Proper bagging will ensure your safety and will comply with recommendations for the proper disposal of infectious waste.

PERITONEAL DIALYSIS WASTE

Peritoneal dialysis patients are often prone to episodes of peritonitis that require hospitalization. If you are involved in the transport of such a patient, it is important to remember that fluid from the catheter or on the dressing could contain hepatitis B virus or cytomegalovirus (CMV). The procedure for handling dressings of and drainage from these patients follows:

1. Disposable gloves should be worn.
2. Dressings should be bagged for incineration.
3. Spillage should be cleaned with a solution of one cup of bleach per gallon of tap water.

PROCEDURE FOR EXPOSURE FOLLOWUP

The procedure for exposure followup can be approached in two ways:

1. Each hospital has an infection control practitioner (ICP). The ICP is aware of all communicable disease cases admitted to the hospital or seen in the emergency department (ED). The ICP also has access to information at other hospitals to which these patients may have been transferred. The ICP would be the ideal person to contact for information. This will centralize information sharing between the hospital and the EMS system.
2. A single member of the ED staff could be designated as the contact person and serve as a liaison between the ICP and the EMS care providers.

Always remember to complete an incident report form to document a possible exposure.

■ COMPLETING A LOG SHEET

Documenting all cleaning routines will help assure quality control. For example, a checklist to record dates and items cleaned can be easily completed and conveniently filed (Fig. 4-1).

Week of _____

Procedure:	Mon.	Tues.	Wed.	Thurs.	Fri.	Sat.	Sun.
Needle and syringe disposal appropriate							
Stretcher cleaned							
Earphones, life pack, walls, and floor washed							
Chair and bench washed							
O_2 dated or changed							
Supply dates checked							
Supplies rotated							
Multi-dose vials in date							

Figure 4-1. Infection control procedure log.

A special procedures form is helpful for recording equipment that has been cleaned, preventive measures that have been used, and names of exposed personnel (Fig. 4-2).

Figure 4-3 is an example of a form devised by the Fairfax County Fire Rescue Service in Fairfax, Virginia and used by the station officer to identify personnel who may require followup treatment for exposure. You can work with the hospital and public health personnel in your area to develop forms to meet your needs.

■ DISPOSAL OF INFECTIOUS WASTE

The handling of infectious waste has become a major issue since 1983, when the Environmental Protection Agency (EPA) issued guidelines for the packaging and disposal of items defined as "infectious."

Items defined as infectious include: needles and sharps, blood and blood products, and dressings from infected wounds and secretions. There are many other items on the list, but these are applicable to your discipline. The concern is that these items could present a hazard if deposited in a landfill. The EPA recommends that either these items be sterilized before being sent to the landfill or that they be incinerated.

The recommended means for packaging these items is listed in Table 4-2. At first these procedures may seem time-consuming, but all changes in routine seem cumbersome at first. Items requiring bagging are generally placed into a "bio-hazard" bag. If bio-hazard bags are not available on your unit, request that they be available in the emergency department.

Hospitals, urgi-centers, and health-care facilities across the country are currently designing their approaches to waste disposal. Take this opportunity to learn from them and share in this process.

Special Procedures   Date: _____
                                                                    Initial

    Suction used and cleaned   _____

    Ambulance used and cleaned   _____

    O_2 used and tubes changed   _____

    Patient in disease alert category   _____

       Specify _____
            Linen bagged   Yes ☐   No ☐
Patient contact surfaces cleaned   Yes ☐   No ☐

Patient name _____

Transported to _____

Patient contacts _____

_____

_____

    Figure 4-2. Special procedures log.

72 ■ CARING FOR YOUR RESCUE VEHICLE, SUPPLIES, AND EQUIPMENT

What was done to prevent/reduce exposure:_____

Decontamination procedures done:_____

_____By Whom?_____

Related medical HX and immunization status of employee(s) if needed:

    Name_____ HX._____

    Name_____ HX._____

Patient's treating ED physician:_____Tel.#_____

Patient's physician (PMD):_____

Location patient dropped off:_____

Name of patient:_____Tel.#_____

Address of patient:_____

Comments:_____

_____

_____

_____

If any questionable areas not addressed in handbook or for further screening and information, contact Infectious Control Practitioner.

Name of ICP_____ Time_____Recommendations_____

_____

_____

Preliminary instructions to employee(s):_____

_____By whom:_____

Recommending treating physician for employee(s) Infectious Disease Physicians Contacted:

    Name_____Date_____Time_____Method_____

Treatment recommendation for employee(s) by Infectious Disease Physician:____

_____

_____

Figure 4-3. Infection control inquiry form. (Fairfax County Fire/Rescue Service)

DISPOSAL OF INFECTIOUS WASTE ■ 73

Person taking report:_____Current date/time:_____

Person initiating inquiry:_____Current date/time:_____

Units involved:_____OIC of incident:_____

Incident number:_____Incident address:_____

Name(s) of exposed Fire & Rescue Department personnel:

    1.   Unit_____Name_____ Hm. Tel.#_____

    2.   Unit_____Name_____ Hm. Tel.#_____

    3.   Unit_____Name_____ Hm. Tel.#_____

    4.   Unit_____Name_____ Hm. Tel.#_____

    5.   Unit_____Name_____ Hm. Tel.#_____

    6.   Unit_____Name_____ Hm. Tel.#_____

    7.   Unit_____Name_____ Hm. Tel.#_____

    8.   Unit_____Name_____ Hm. Tel.#_____

Suspected Disease (reported lab data?) (be as specific as possible):_____

_____

_____

Patient contact time: Start_____ Completed_____

Type of exposure: Via what route? (blood, body fluid or secretion)_____

_____

_____

Describe details of exposure: (area of body contact)_____

_____

_____

Conditions of exposure: (Locations - confined spaces, etc.)_____

_____

_____

Figure 4-3. Continued

■ Table 4-2. PACKAGING INFECTIOUS WASTE

Discard *sharps* directly into impervious, rigid, puncture proof containers
Discard *liquid* infectious wastes in capped or tightly stoppered bottles or flasks
For other infectious wastes, use plastic bags that are
  Seamless
  Impervious
  Tear resistant
  Red or orange in color
  Strong enough to remain intact during handling and treatment

Blood Spills

As mentioned previously, blood spills can be hazardous. Because the hepatitis B virus can survive for long periods on surfaces, cleaning blood-contaminated areas is crucial and should be performed before any other vehicle areas are cleaned.

POLICY
To remove possible hepatitis B virus, carry out priority cleaning when handling blood.

PROCEDURE
First clean all areas covered with blood. Wear disposable gloves. Dilute Clorox or household bleach, using a 1:10 solution—1 part bleach to 10 parts water (Fig. 4-4 and Fig. 4-5).

■ REUSING DISPOSABLES

Most medical personnel, including those involved in EMS systems, are working actively to reduce health-care costs. In this attempt to lower costs, many EMS systems throughout the United States are reprocessing disposable supplies. In March 1984 a conference was held in Washington, DC to discuss the reuse of disposable medical devices. The issues addressed included the economic, legal, ethical, and scientific implications of such procedures.

A major concern at this conference was whether a disposable product could be reprocessed and still be considered sterile

REUSING DISPOSABLES ■ 75

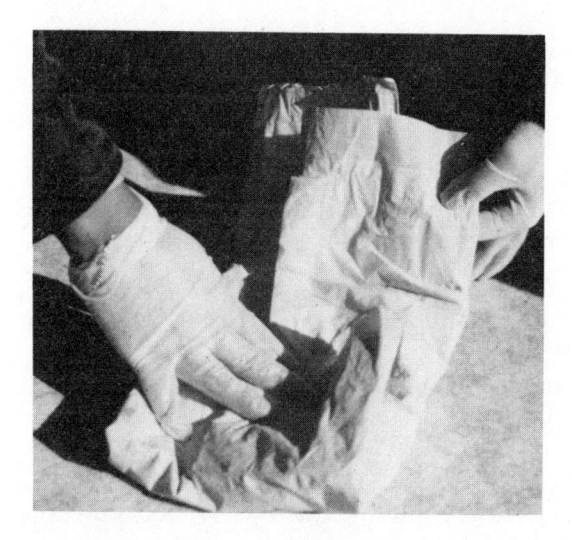

Figure 4-4. Cleaning blood spills using gloves.

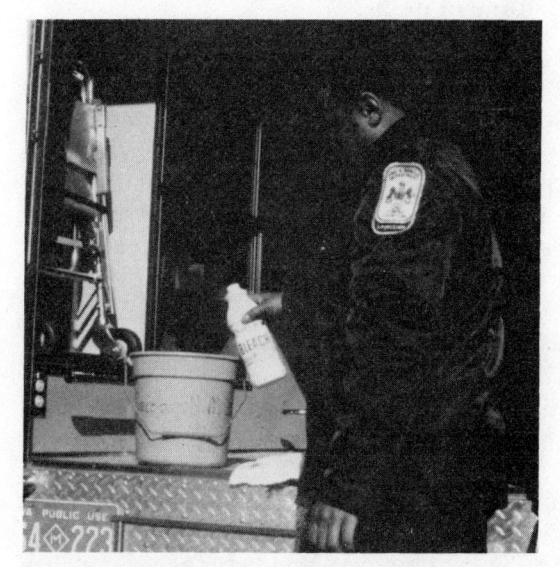

Figure 4-5. Diluting bleach.

and functional. Documented cases reveal that patients have sustained injuries following the use of reprocessed disposable items. These cases resulted in liability cases with awarded settlements.[3]

If your system is currently reprocessing disposable items such as oral airways, tongue depressors, and the like, or if your system is planning to reprocess these items, consider the following points:

1. Toxicity—Many disposable items absorb the chemicals used in reprocessing. If traces of these chemicals remain on the items, the patient may be affected adversely.
2. Sterility—If the item was originally used as a sterile item, such as an endotracheal tube, the reprocessing procedure and packaging should ensure sterility.[4,5]
3. Proper functioning—The manufacturer is responsible for the item's performance. However, if you reprocess the item, this responsibility becomes yours.
4. Physical appearance of the item—Reprocessing may alter the item physically, which may not be visible.
5. Reprocessing creates additional hazards in the workplace and increased handling of items.

Legal liability is an important issue. If your system is considering reprocessing, carefully consider and examine packaging statements, warranties, and regulations. Currently, regulating agencies such as the Food & Drug Administration (FDA) state that single-use or disposable items should not be reused.[3,6,7]

Is this process cost-effective? In fact, costs may actually increase, taking into account solutions, labor, and potential liability. Therefore, the general recommendation is to avoid reprocessing at least until procedures have been tested and guidelines and recommendations have been sanctioned.

■ CLEANING AND MAINTAINING TRAINING MANIKINS

Guidelines for decontaminating Annie were first published by the CDC in 1978, but were not usually followed because they were time-consuming. Now, however, medical personnel are concerned about contracting infections from training manikins. And even though the Annie manikin never has been shown as a source of infection, the possibility of this being the case may exist. In 1983, as a result of this concern, the CDC, the American Heart Association, and the Committee on Emergency Care decided to discuss the issue and develop new guidelines for decontaminating training manikins. Based on the original guidelines, the new guidelines include the following considerations:

1. Inform students in advance that training sessions will involve close physical contact with their fellow students.
2. Students should not participate in training sessions if they have the following conditions: skin lesions on hands or in oral areas; blood positive for hepatitis B surface antigen; upper respiratory tract infections; AIDS; have had exposure to or have an active infection.
3. If more than one CPR manikin is used, students should work in pairs. Each pair should practice on one manikin only.
4. CPR instructors should advocate thorough handwashing procedures, as well as maintain clean manikins.
5. Routinely inspect manikins for cracks or tears in plastic surfaces that would make thorough cleaning difficult.
6. Wash manikins' clothes and hair monthly or whenever visibly soiled.[8]

Decontaminating Manikins After Each Student Use

1. After each student uses a manikin, wipe the manikin's mouth and lips with a 2"X2" gauze pad dampened with a solution of 1:10 bleach and water or 70% isopropyl alchohol. The surface should remain wet for at least 30 seconds before it is wiped dry (Fig. 4-6).
2. If you are using a protective face shield, change it before each student.

Reducing Contamination During Two-Rescuer CPR Instruction

1. During two-rescuer CPR instruction, disinfecting the manikin after each student uses it is not practical. To reduce the

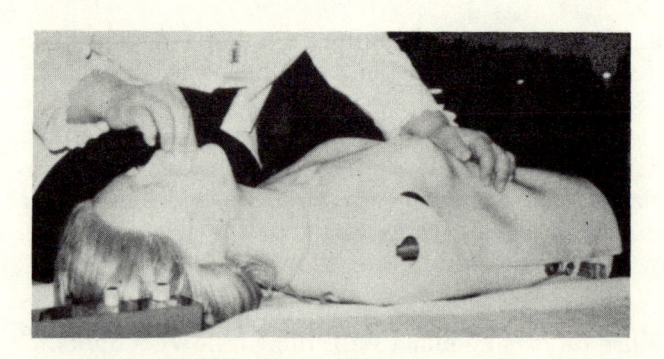

Figure 4-6. Cleaning a manikin.

possibility of transmitting disease during this exercise, have the second student who is taking over ventilations just simulate the ventilations. This variation from normal practice is recommended by the American Red Cross and the American Heart Association.[8]

2. When a student uses his or her finger to sweep foreign matter out of a manikin's mouth, contamination could occur from previous students' saliva. Also, saliva could contaminate the manikin. The finger sweep that is used when practicing the obstructed airway procedure either should be simulated or should be performed on a manikin whose airway was decontaminated before the procedure and will be decontaminated after the procedure.[8]

Postclass Decontaminating Procedures

1. Disassemble manikin as directed by manufacturer.
2. Thoroughly wash all external and internal surfaces, as well as reusable protective face shields, with warm soapy water and brushes.
3. Rinse all surfaces with fresh water.
4. Wet all surfaces with a sodium hypochlorite solution (1:10 bleach to water) for 10 minutes. Use a freshly made solution and discard after using.
5. Rinse with fresh water and dry all surfaces. Rinsing with

alcohol will help dry internal surfaces and destroy bacterial or fungal pathogens.[8,9]

■ SUPPLY ROTATION

POLICY
Supplies should be checked daily.

PROCEDURE
Stock items should be checked daily for expiration dates. The stock with the shortest time to expiration should be kept forward. Expired stock should be removed and disposed of appropriately.

■ STETHOSCOPES

POLICY
The stethoscope is often ignored as a potential carrier of bacteria. One study shows that colonization of the bell, or diaphragm, may occur. *Staphylococcus aureus, Serratia,* and *Pseudomonas* organisms were isolated from 8% of the stethoscopes in the study.[10]

PROCEDURE
As stethoscopes may harbor pathogenic organisms, they should be cleaned after they are used in examining infected patients (i.e., with skin lesions or drainage). Probably they should be cleaned on a daily basis.

■ MULTI-DOSE VIALS

The Centers for Disease Control state that a multi-dose vial can be considered safe to use if it is currently in date and if it has been stored according to the manufacturer's recommendation on the package insert. Studies have shown that vials have not grown bacteria after 90 days of use. Here is an opportunity for your service to save some money by not having to purchase single-use vials.

POLICY

Vial expiration dates should serve as a guide for maximum storage time. A vial should be discarded if obvious contamination is apparent, if it is cracked, or if it has not been stored in accordance with the directions on the label. Area hospital guidelines for vial disposal should be used.[11]

PROCEDURE

In keeping with the policy of many hospitals, a 24-hour limit may be imposed on all open multi-dose vials (*i.e.*, sterile water for injection). Otherwise, all vials should be dated when opened and are usually discarded after 30 days.

■ NEEDLE AND SYRINGE DISPOSAL

The new recommendations for disposal of needles and syringes came about in an effort to reduce needle-stick injuries, thus reducing risks to health-care providers. Research has shown that aerosolization takes place when needles are cut or bent, thereby creating the risk of inhalation of droplets. The old system (Fig. 4-7) should be replaced by one of the new systems available. There are many to choose from. Figure 4-8 shows one of the types of containers available.

Note that the recapping of needles also is not recommended. This is when most needle sticks occur, especially when recapping in the back of a moving vehicle. As a container may not be readily available in your unit, styrofoam may help with needle placement until a container is available (Fig. 4-9).

POLICY

All needles and syringes should be disposed of in a manner that complies with EPA recommendations for the disposal of hazardous waste.

NEEDLE AND SYTRINGE DISPOSAL ■ 81

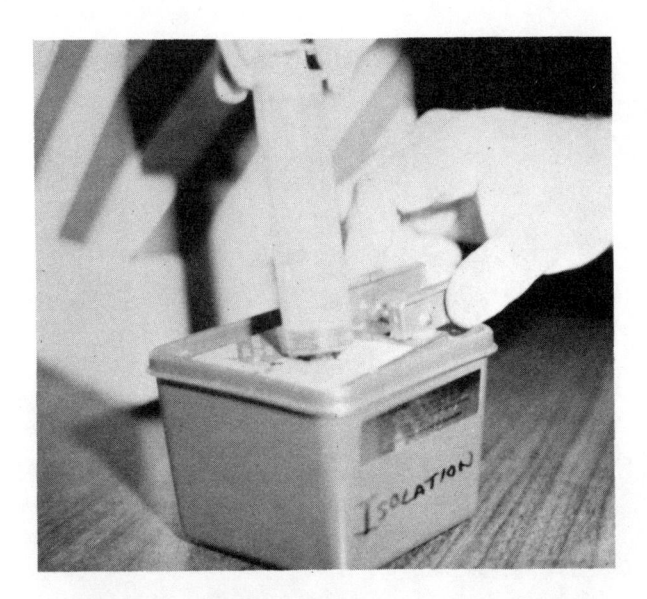

Figure 4-7. Needle disposal.

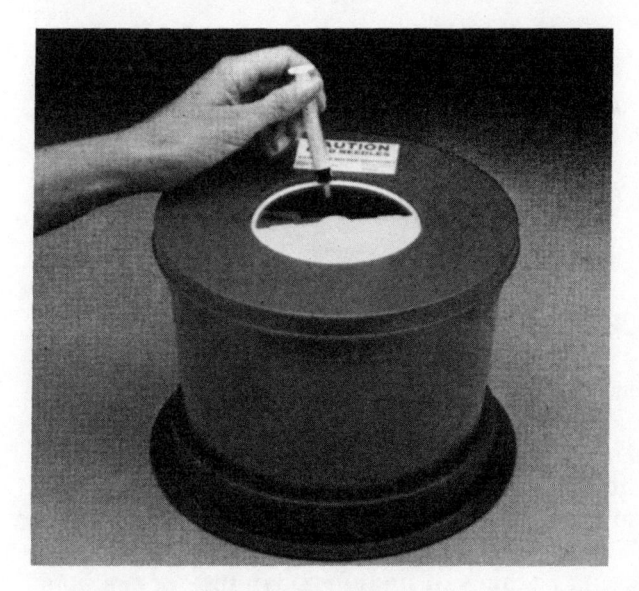

Figure 4-8. Needle container.

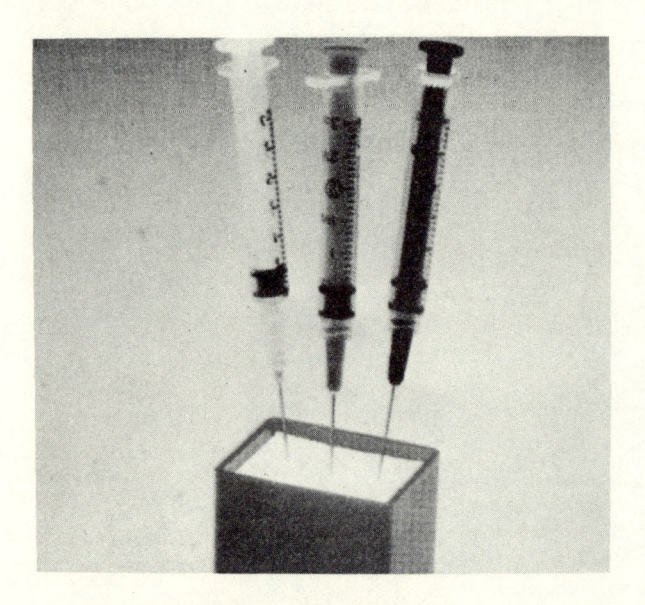

Figure 4-9. Needles placed in styrofoam.

PROCEDURE

Needles should not be cut off, nor should the hubs be cut off the syringes. Cut needles can result in the aerosolization of blood or medication. Needles should not be recapped, since this is when most needle sticks occur. The entire unit should be placed in a puncture-proof container. When filled, the container should be incinerated.

■ RESPIRATORY THERAPY EQUIPMENT

O_2 Setups (Humidifiers)

If you are still using O_2 humidifiers, here are some considerations. First, the CDC has determined that there is a very small chance that these humidifiers could become a source of infection in the hospital. The situation is a bit different, however, in your vehicle. If you are using the wall suction apparatus, for example, there is a chance of contamination through aerosolization. Therefore, if disposable O_2 humidifiers are used, they should be dated when opened and discarded after 5 days.[12] Ideally, they should be a patient charge item and should be changed after each patient.

Current studies on the benefits offered patients by O_2 humidification state that the only benefit would be if you had a long transport time—2 hours or longer—so EMS personnel in many areas can delete this item from their inventories.[13]

POLICY
Once the seal is broken and the system is opened, the setup should be changed in 5 days. O_2 humidification is only of value for cases with a long transport time (2 hours or longer).

PROCEDURE
When an O_2 humidifier is hooked up, it should be dated. The unit should be discarded after 5 days,[9] or it may be handled as a patient charge item and be changed after each patient.

Ambu Bags

POLICY
Ambu bags should be sterilized after each use.

PROCEDURE
Disassemble equipment, clean with soap and water, and place in a cold liquid sterilization solution for 20 minutes. Then air dry for at least 1 hour (Fig. 4-10). One-time use bags are available.

Suction Equipment

Handling suction secretions can pose a risk, so you need to handle them with care. The vehicle wall suction apparatus is an unfiltered system. This means that when you are running the system you are aerosolizing the secretions you are sunctioning. Disposable systems, that have filters built into the canister unit, are available on the market. These disposable units are designed to meet EPA guidelines for disposing of liquid waste—they can be capped following use and bagged for disposal. The receptacles

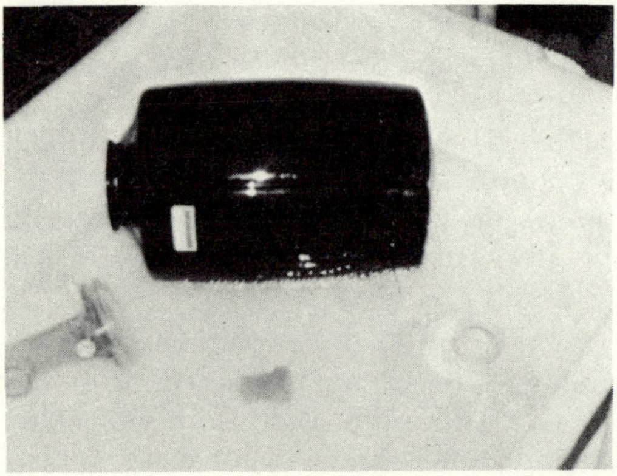

Figure 4-10. Cleaning respiratory equipment.

are a permanent part of the vehicle and are furnished by the companies. The liners slide down inside the canister and, when filled, they can be capped and easily removed (Fig. 4-11).

If you are using your wall suction unit, it should be disinfected after each use. The tubing needs to be flushed with disinfectant solution and allowed to air dry. The contents of the canister should be carefully poured out at drain level (Fig. 4-12), which will decrease the chance of splashing.

POLICY
Suction equipment should be cleaned after each use.

PROCEDURE
Disposable equipment should be bagged and set aside for incineration. Nondisposable sets should be cleaned as follows:

1. The bottle should be emptied carefully so that splashing does not occur.
2. The bottle should be washed out with a germicidal or viricidal agent and air dried.
3. The latex tubing should be cleaned as the bottle is cleaned and allowed to air dry[14] (Fig. 4-13).

RESPIRATORY THERAPY EQUIPMENT ■ 85

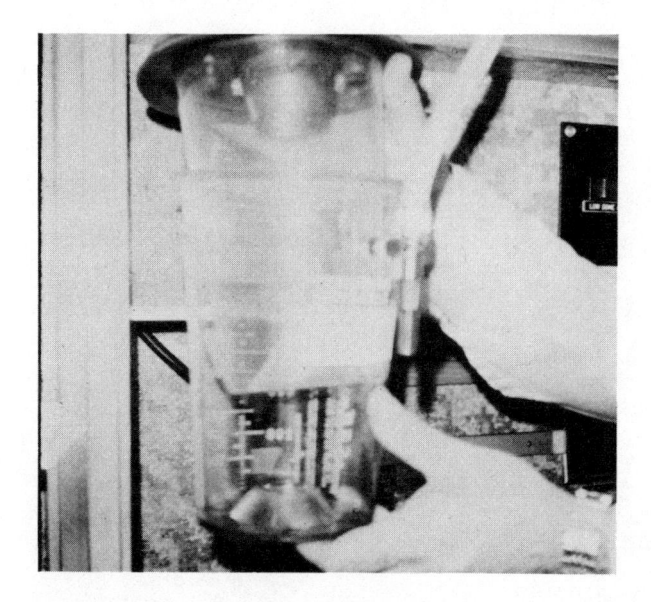

Figure 4-11. Suction equipment.

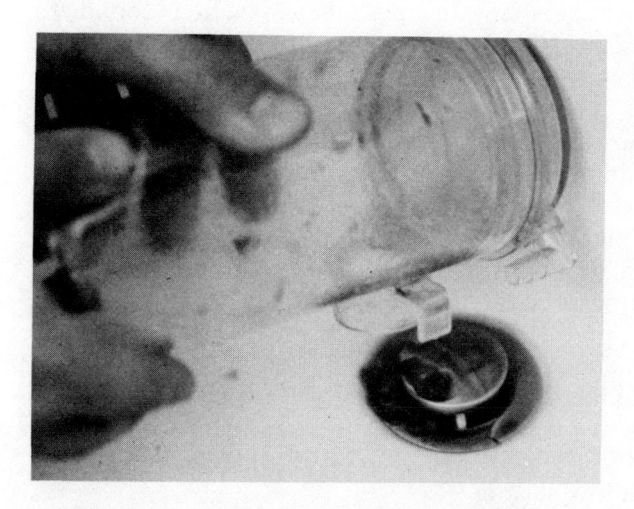

Figure 4-12. Pouring from canister.

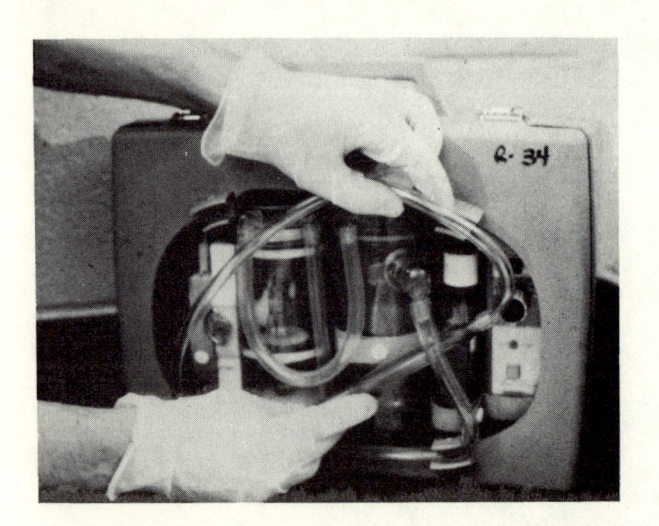

Figure 4-13. Tubing.

ANTISHOCK TROUSERS

POLICY
Antishock trousers should be cleaned when soiled to remove blood and secretions.

PROCEDURE
The procedure for cleaning this equipment is dependent on whether the bladders are removable or nonremovable.

Removable Bladders. Remove and close air chambers. Wipe with a cloth dampened with an antiseptic soap and detergent. Rinse with warm water and allow to air dry. DO NOT MACHINE WASH OR MACHINE DRY.

Non-removable bladders. *Outer Garment*—Hand or machine wash at a medium temperature setting, with a detergent soap. DO NOT WASH WITH OTHER ITEMS. Air dry or machine dry at a low setting.

To sterilize outer garments, or those without removable

bladders, gas sterilize or use a cold liquid sterilization solution. Antishock trousers should never be stored wet or damp. Never use drycleaning solutions or chemical solvents. Do not bleach, do not boil or steam sterilize, do not iron or press.[15]

■ IV BAGS

If the outer bag is removed from your IV, are the contents sterile? Yes—as long as you are comfortable with the fact that you have not added a medication or the tab has not been removed—it is indeed sterile. It is up to your service to make its own determination about whether these bags need to be thrown out or not. Saving them for reuse can be a cost-saving measure.

■ References

1. Garner JS, Simmons BP: CDC Guidelines for isolation precautions in hospitals. Infect Control 4:249–257, 1983
2. West KW: Infection Control Recommendation for Rescue Vehicles. 1982
3. Holzer JF: Product liability. Assoc. Advancement Med Instrument, 44–47, 1983
4. Benson DW: Disposable endoliacheal tubes: How safe to reuse?, JAMA, 244(15): 1721, 1980
5. Belani KG: Reuse of disposable endotracheal tubes. JAMA, 245(9):922, 1981
6. Barnes, A: Reuse and JCAH accreditation, Journal HSPD, 2(4):44–52, 1984
7. FDA Reuse of Medical Disposable Devices: Compliance Guide 7124.23. Silver Spring, Bureau of Medical Devices, 1977
8. Recommendations for decontaminating manikins used in cardiopulmonary resuscitation training: 1983 update. Infect Control, 5(8):399–401, 1984
9. Cavagnolo RZ: Inactivation of herpes virus on CPR manikins utilizing a currently recommended disinfecting procedure. Infect Control, 6:456–458, 1985
10. The stethoscope: A vector of infection? Infect Control, 4(4):189, 1983

11. Infection risks of multiple dose vials examined. Hospital Infect Control, 157-159, December 1981
12. Singer H: Respiratory therapy. Score, 4-6, Summer 1977
13. Brown T, Marsch C: Dry vs humidified low flow oxygen. Respir Care, 1031, October 1984
14. Centers for Disease Control: The control of pulmonary infection associated with suctioning. Quarterly Report, 1981
15. The Jobst Institute: Personal Communication, October 1983

Infection Control Program Costs 5

Perhaps you feel that organizing an infection control program may increase the expenses of your emergency medical service system, considering supplies and administrative costs involved in implementing the recommended activities. Before discussing cost, however, let's review the advantages of the program.

Establishing an employee health maintenance program would determine more effectively existing health problems of new medical personnel. Records documenting illnesses contracted on the job would be more readily available, unnecessary absences may be eliminated, and preventive measures may reduce disability claims.[1] Systems that offer immunization and preventive medicine programs often are rewarded with a decrease in insurance premiums. Insurance premium discounts should be investigated.

Furthermore, clearly written policies and procedures help to reduce potential liability situations in your EMS system. This reduction should be especially noticeable in areas regarding work restrictions, job-related illnesses, and exposure situations. With increasing occupational health risks for medical personnel, contracted illnesses are resulting in litigation and financial expense for many health-care workers.[2,3] Also, a well-defined health program may have a positive effect on employee morale and reduce employee turnover. Retraining and orienting requires time and money, but reducing turnover ultimately saves money.

Finally, improved cleaning procedures will protect both medical personnel and patients. At present, 2% to 15% of all hospital admissions develop hospital-acquired or nosocomial infections.[4] These infections often result from actual treatment procedures, such as IV placement, respiratory therapy measures, surgery, and antibiotic therapy. When evaluating these nosocomial infections, procedures that are performed during the prehospital care phase must be considered. In the past 10 years, emergency care in the field has advanced, and invasive procedures have been performed under difficult conditions. However, medical personnel must attempt to control the situation and protect the patient.

The cleaning recommendations listed in this handbook have been researched and are recommended nationwide. Note that the guidelines presented are often referred to as the standards for care of or duty to patients. In essence, an effective infection control program can reduce the incidence of legal liability by adhering to documented standards.

An example of a situation that illustrates potential liability is as follows: A hospital infection-control nurse identifies several patients with respiratory infections all caused by the same organism. An in depth review of the cases yields two common factors in all of the patients. Each patient had been brought to the hospital by the same rescue squad, and each patient had had ventilation assistance during the transport. The bag–mask resuscitator was cultured, and it grew the same organism that had infected the patients. The EMS personnel responsible for this unit did not sterilize the bag–mask resuscitator after each use, as is currently recommended.

Cleaning supply costs can be reduced by in depth product evaluation: Does the product perform effectively, and is the cost comparable to other, similar products? Does the manufacturer offer volume discounts? Can your system purchase supplies through the hospital's group buying service? Do hospitals share supplies with your service? Each of these approaches can result in a significant reduction in the cost of supplies.

Each EMS system should evaluate all recommendations and their appropriateness to its system. The ultimate objective of implementation of cleaning and aseptic procedures is the reduction of morbidity and mortality.

Throughout the United States, hospitals are attempting to reduce costs and improve public relations with the community. If you feel that the infection-control program presented in this handbook is feasible, approach the facilities you serve and ascertain how combining efforts may help reduce your costs and utilize your services more effectively.

References

1. Williams WW: CDC guidelines for infection control in hospital personnel. Infect Control, 4(4):327–349, 1983
2. Booker vs Duke Medical Center. 297 NC 458 256 SE, 2nd 1989 (1979)
3. Bell v Industrial Vangas. 637 P 2d, 266 (Cal 1981)
4. Doschner FD: Practical aspects for cost reduction in hospital infection control. Infect Control, 12–15, 1984

EMS–Hospital Relations: Establishing a Contact Person

6

Communication between your EMS system and the hospital(s) you serve is crucial for organizing and maintaining an effective infection-control program and it probably will also help ease personnel apprehension. Two approaches to establishing a contact person can be taken. The first approach involves selecting one person in the hospital emergency department who will answer questions and who will notify medical personnel working in field situations when they have been exposed to communicable patients. Designating only one person to handle these responsibilities will assure relaying accurate information. Communication models have stressed that the more people involved in communication, the greater the chances of misinterpreting the information.[1]

The second approach involves utilizing your hospital's infection control practitioner (ICP) as your contact person. Because ICPs are knowledgeable about infectious and communicable diseases, they are able to screen medical personnel in exposure situations, as well as answer their questions and advise them regarding such exposure. ICP personnel may include registered nurses, licensed practical nurses, or medical technologists who are specifically trained in infectious and communicable diseases. A recent national survey revealed that over 80% of the ICPs are registered nurses.[2] ICPs are logical choices for contact persons because they routinely identify and report to the Public Health Department patients with infectious and communicable diseases who have been admitted to their hospitals or who have been seen or treated in their emergency departments. Figure 6-1 is a conceptual model that illustrates how utilizing ICPs will facilitate accurate followup communication.

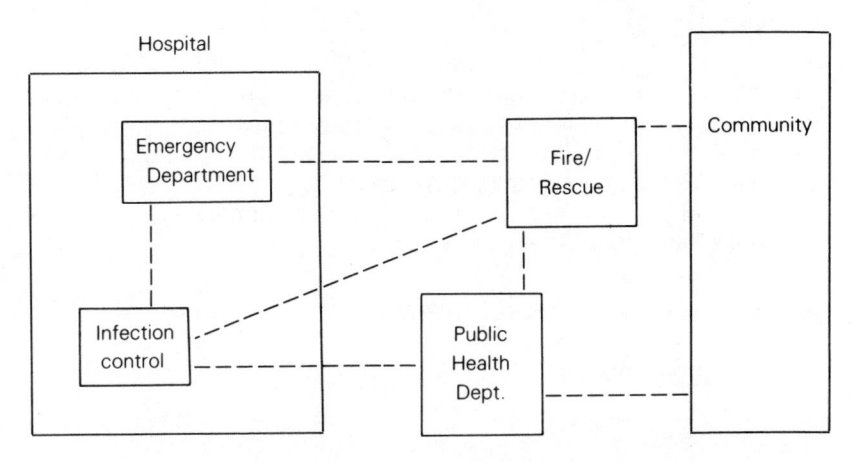

Figure 6-1. Hospital–community interaction conceptual model.

After the ICP reports to the Public Health Department, the department contacts people in the community who may have been exposed to the infectious patient. Traditionally, fire and rescue personnel have been omitted from this service, but they should be brought into the process. With this approach to improving communication in the medical community, EMS personnel easily can be included in the relay of information.

Other ICP job responsibilities include educating hospital personnel regarding infectious diseases and controlling infection. This may be another resource for your department.[3] Perhaps your hospital's ICP can conduct training sessions or supply educational materials for your personnel.

If you are interested in developing this network, schedule a meeting with the ICPs in your area hospitals. Discuss your needs and concerns and ask how ICPs can help you meet those needs. Because hospitals today are making many changes anyway, you may find that administrative and medical personnel will be very receptive and, in fact, anxious to improve hospital–community relations.

References

1. Axnick KJ, Yarbrough M: Infection control: An Integrated Approach, pp 30–41. St. Louis, CV Mosby, 1984
2. A national task analysis of infection control practictioners, 1982. Am J Infect Control 12(2):88–95, 1984
3. Wenzel RP: Handbook of Hospital Acquired Infections, pp. 19–34. Boca Raton, CRC Press, 1981

Appendix

■ Infectious Disease Quick Reference

The first section of this appendix lists all of the infectious diseases in an alphabetical quick reference format. The protective measures recommended for each disease are in both written and picture format. The key below describes the picture symbols used.

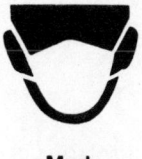

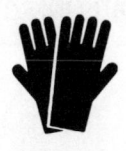

Mask   Gloves   Handwashing

■ AIDS (ACQUIRED IMMUNE DEFICIENCY SYNDROME)

Mode of transmission: Contact with blood or bodily secretions or sexual contact.
Protective measures: Wear disposable gloves when in contact with blood or body fluids.
  Wash hands following patient care, even if gloves were used.

Use portable CPR equipment (disposable airway and ambu bag), whenever possible.
Purchasing AIDS suits or AIDS kits is not recommended and is an additional expense.
Wear disposable gowns *only* when clothing may be soiled with blood or body fluids.

■ CHICKENPOX (VARICELLA ZOSTER)

Mode of transmission: Spread by droplets and airborne secretions from the respiratory tract.
Protective measures: Wear disposable mask and gloves.

■ CMV (CYTOMEGALOVIRUS INFECTION)

Mode of transmission: Direct contact with secretions from cervix, or with semen, blood, feces, saliva, and urine.
Preventive measures: Wear disposable gloves. Use good handwashing technique when in contact with secretions.

■ GONORRHEA

Mode of transmission: Sexual contact, including oral–genital contact, with an infected person.
Preventive measures: When in contact with secretions of the genital tract, wear disposable gloves and use good handwashing technique.

■ HEPATITIS A

Mode of transmission: Contact with stool, blood, or urine of an infected individual.
Methods for protection: Handwashing following contact with excretions, or use disposable gloves.

■ HEPATITIS B (SERUM HEPATITIS)

Mode of transmission: Blood, mucous membranes (saliva, sputum), sexual contact.
Protective measures: Wear disposable gloves when in contact with blood, saliva, or sputum. Use good handwashing technique.

■ HERPES SIMPLEX TYPE 1 (COLD SORE, FEVER BLISTER)

Mode of transmission: Direct contact with lesions or with oral mucous membranes.
Protective measures: Wear disposable gloves when in contact with lesions or mucous membranes. Use good handwashing technique.

■ HERPES SIMPLEX TYPE 2 (GENITAL HERPES)

Mode of transmission: Direct sexual contact with lesions or skin to lesion contact. This virus enters through breaks in the skin;

it is not airborne and can not be contracted from toilet seats, pools, hot tubs, or sheets.
Protective measures: Wear disposable gloves when in contact with lesions. Use good handwashing technique.

■ HERPES WHITLOW (HERPES SIMPLEX INFECTION OF THE FINGER)

Mode of transmission: Virus enters through breaks in the skin after contact with oral or tracheal secretions of patient shedding herpes virus.
Protective measures: Wear disposable gloves on both hands when in contact with oral or tracheal secretions. Use good handwashing technique.

■ HERPES ZOSTER (SHINGLES)

Mode of transmission: Direct contact with infected vesicles.
Protective measures: Wear disposable gloves when in contact with draining lesions. Use good handwashing technique.

■ LICE (PEDICULOSIS)

Mode of transmission:

Head and body louse: Close contact with infected persons or their personal items, such as scarves, hats, combs, and furniture.
Crab louse: Sexual contact, bedding, or clothing (rarely by toilet seat).

Protective measures: Wear disposable gloves when possible.

■ MALARIA (JUNGLE FEVER)

Mode of transmission: Bite of a female anopheles mosquito. Can be contracted through blood transfusion.
Protective measures: Risks are minimal to EMS personnel who care for patients with a history of malaria. Even if you sustain a needle-stick injury, the chances of contracting the disease are still very low.

■ MEASLES—RUBELLA (GERMAN)

Mode of transmission: By droplets or direct contact with nasopharyngeal secretions, blood, urine, and stool of an infected individual. Can be contracted by fetus from pregnant woman who has contracted the disease.
Protective measures: Wear disposable gloves when handling secretions or excretions. Mask the patient or yourself.

■ MEASLES—RUBEOLA (RED)

Mode of transmission: By droplets or direct contact with nasopharyngeal secretions or urine of an infected individual.
Protective measures: Wear disposable gloves and mask when in close contact with secretions of the mouth, nose, and throat, or with urine.

■ MENINGITIS (BACTERIAL)

Mode of transmission: Direct contact with discharges from nose or throat.
Protective measures: Mask the patient or yourself.

■ MENINGITIS (VIRAL, ASEPTIC)

Mode of transmission: Droplets.
Protective measures: Since diagnosis is unknown at the time of your patient contact, mask the patient or yourself.

■ MUMPS (INFECTIOUS PAROTITIS)

Mode of transmission: Direct contact with saliva.
Protective measures: Disposable gloves when in contact with oral secretions. Good handwashing.

■ PERTUSSIS (WHOOPING COUGH)

Mode of transmission: Contact with infected respiratory secretions.
Protective measures: Wear a mask when in contact with secretions of the mouth, the nose, and the throat.

■ PULMONARY TUBERCULOSIS

Mode of transmission: Airborne droplets, primarily during sneezing, coughing, speaking, or singing. Prolonged contact with an active TB case is most significant. Contact with thick, coughed-up sputum is also significant.
Protective measures: Mask the patient, if possible. If patient masking not possible, mask yourself. Rapid fresh air ventilation, as available in your vehicle.

■ RABIES (HYDROPHOBIA)

Mode of transmission: Direct contact with saliva of an infected animal. The virus may enter any area of broken skin. Human-to-human transmission has not been documented.
Protective measures: Wear disposable gloves. Use good handwashing technique when in contact with saliva.

■ SALMONELLA

Mode of transmission: Ingesting contaminated food or water. Contact with infected feces.
Protective measures: Wear disposable gloves. Use good handwashing technique when in contact with stools.

■ SCABIES

Mode of transmission: Skin-to-skin contact. Extensive hands-on contact is usually required for transmission to occur.
Protective measures: Wear disposable gloves when possible. Use thorough handwashing technique.

■ SYPHILIS (PRIMARY SYPHILIS)

Mode of transmission: Direct sexual contact or blood of an infected person.

Protective measures: Wear disposable gloves and use good handwashing technique when in contact with lesion or blood.

■ Glossary

Aerosalization. Atomized particles suspended in the air, which create droplets.
Airborne infection. An infection transferred from one person to another, without direct contact between them, by means of droplets of moisture containing the infectious agent.
Antigen. A substance that brings about the formation of protective antibodies.
Antibody. A protein that gives immunity (immunoglobulin). Antibodies are natives of the body; many are present at birth.
Bacteria. Any microorganisms of the class Schizomycetes (there are three forms, which vary in size). May produce poisonous substances called toxins.
Baseline. A documented foundation to build on (an initial record).
Communicable disease. An illness caused by a specific infectious agent that is transmitted to a susceptible host.
Cytomegalovirus. A member of a group of viruses closely related to the herpes viruses.
Dialysis. The separation of substances, one from another, in solution.
Disinfectant. A chemical that kills infectious agents.
Droplet. A minute particle of moisture expelled by talking, sneezing, or coughing, thereby transmitting from one person to another.
Dysuria. Pain on urination.
Eruption. The sudden appearance of lesions on the skin.
Exposure. Subjection to an infectious agent.
Fungus. A vegetable cellular organism that lives on organic matter; a spongelike growth on the body that resembles fungi.
Germicidal. An agent that is destructive to germs.
Hepatitis. A viral infection that causes damage to and destruction of liver cells, resulting in inflammation and death of cells. Regeneration of cells usually occurs. In severe cases, nodules separated by connective tissue can lead to cirrhosis.

Icterus. Yellow coloration of the tissues, membranes, and secretions with bile pigment. See **jaundice**.
Immune system. The body's defense against bacteria and viruses.
Incubation period. The interval between exposure to an infection and the appearance of the first symptom.
Infection. The invasion of tissues by pathogenic microorganisms.
Isolation. The separation of infected persons from others to prevent spread of an infectious agent.
Jaundice. Marked by yellow skin and sclerae due to changes in liver cells or obstruction that causes the bile pigment, bilirubin, to be diffused into the blood. Also known as icterus.
Lesion. An alteration (structural or functional), usually on the skin, due to disease.
Louse (lice). A small, wingless, flattened insect.
Meningitis. Inflammation of the membranes of the spinal cord or brain.
Mode of transmission. The manner by which an infectious agent is spread.
Mononucleosis (mono). An illness characterized by an increase in the number of monocytes appearing in the blood or tissues.
Peritoneal dialysis. Dialysis performed through the peritoneal cavity. Can be either continuous or intermittent.
PPD (purified protein derivitive). A screening test for tuberculosis.
Preicteric. Before jaundice.
Pruritus. Severe itching, sometimes caused by irritation of cutaneous nerves by retained bile sales, or bilirubin, diffused into the blood.
Scabies. A mite.
Shedding. Casting off or throwing off, as with viruses.
Symptomatic treatment. Treatment of specific symptoms of a disease that can not cure the disease.
Tetanus. An infectious disease characterized by extreme stiffness of the body.
Toxic hepatitis. Caused by exposure to certain poisons (carbon

tetrachloride) or drugs (sulfonamides), or by respiratory disturbances.

Vaccine. A preparation administered to induce immunity in the recipient.

Viral. Caused by a virus.

Viricidal. An agent that is destructive to viruses.

Index

Numbers followed by an *f* indicate a figure; *t* following a page number indicates a table.

Acu-dyne, 12t
Acyclovir, in herpes infections, 59
Aerosolization, 82, 83, 101
AIDS (acquired immune deficiency syndrome), 46–50
  exposure followup, 50
  guidelines for medical personnel, 48
  hepatitis B immunization and, 4
  protective (preventive) measures, 49, 50, 95, 96
  "safe" sex recommendations, 48
  symptoms, 47, 50
  transmission, 47, 49, 95
Alcare, 12t
Alcohol
  for disinfecting rescue vehicle/equipment, 66t
  for IV site preparation, 13
Alcohol foam agents, for handwashing, 12t
Ambu bag, sterilization of, 83, 84f
Ammonium compounds, quaternary, for disinfecting rescue vehicle/equipment, 67t
"Annie." *See* CPR manikin

Antibody
  definition of, 101
  to hepatitis B core antigen, 21t, 22
  to hepatitis B surface antigen, 21t, 22
Antigen, definition of, 101
Antiseptics, for IV site preparation, 13, 14t
  application procedure, 13, 15f
Antishock trousers, cleaning, 86–87
Autoinfection, herpes simplex, 59

Bacteria
  definition of, 101
  meningitis from, 29
Bar soaps, for handwashing, 12t
Beatdine, 12t
Blood spills, cleaning procedure, 74, 75f

Cal-stat, 12t
Catheter
  introduction and stabilization of, site preparation for, 13, 14t, 15f
  peritoneal, 10, 11f
    protective (preventive) measures for, 10–11

107

INDEX

Centers for Disease Control (CDC), guidelines for medical personnel caring for AIDS patient, 48
Chest x-ray, for EMS personnel, 1
"Chevron" method, of needle stabilization, 13
Chickenpox (varicella), 40–42, 42f
  in adults, 41
  in EMS personnel, work status, 5
  exposure followup, 42
  immunization, 41t
  protective (preventive) measures, 41, 96
  symptoms, 41
  transmission, 40, 41, 96
Chlorhexidine gluconate, for handwashing, 12t
Chlorine, for disinfecting rescue vehicle equipment, 66t, 67
Chlorox, for cleaning blood spills, 74, 75f
Cold sore. See Herpes simplex, oral infection
Communicable disease, 16–64. See also specific diseases
  AIDS, 46–50, 95–96
  chickenpox, 40–42, 96
  cytomegalovirus (CMV) infection, 50–51, 96
  definition of, 101
  exposure to
    department policy regarding, 6
    risk of infection from, formula for determining, 6
    during transport of patient, 69
  gonorrhea, 44–45, 96
  hepatitis, 19–28, 96
  herpes viruses, 52–61, 97
    simplex, 53–59
    zoster, 60–61

impetigo, 36
lice, 51–52, 98
malaria, 31–32, 98
measles, 37–39, 98
meningitis, 28–31, 99
mumps, 40
pertussis (whooping cough), 42–44, 99
protective measures, 95–100. See also specific diseases
rabies, 32, 34, 35t, 99
salmonella infection, 34–36, 100
scabies, 52, 100
sexually transmitted, 44–52. See also specific diseases
syphilis, 45–46, 100
transporting a patient with
  cleaning and disinfecting rescue vehicle, 68
  exposure followup for EMS personnel, 69
  infectious waste disposal, 68
tuberculosis, 16–19, 99
Congenital cytomegalovirus infection, 50
Congenital rubella syndrome, 3, 38
Conjunctivitis, in EMS personnel, work status, 4
CPR manikin
  cleaning and maintenance, 76–79
  decontaminating after class, 78
  decontaminating after each student use, 77, 78f
  guidelines for use and care, 77
  reducing contamination during 2-person CPR instruction, 77–78
Crabs. See Lice
Cytomegalovirus infection, 50–51
  exposure followup, 51
  protective (preventive) measures, 51, 96

symptoms, 51
transmission, 96

Delta agent, 23
Dialysis patient
  peritoneal, 10–11, 102
    infectious waste disposal, 69
    protective (preventive)
      measures, 10–11
Diarrhea
  in EMS personnel, work status
    and, 4
  in patient, protective
    (preventive) measures, 10
Diphtheria, immunization, 2
Disposable supplies, reuse of, 74, 76
Disinfectants
  definition of, 101
  guidelines for use, 66–67t
Draining wound. See Wounds, draining
Droplets, 16, 101

EMS-hospital relations, 92–94
EMS personnel
  exposure to communicable
    disease. See also
    Communicable disease;
    specific diseases
    risk of infection from,
      formula for determining, 6
    during transport of patient,
      followup protocol for, 69
  health record, 1–4
    immunizations, 2–4. See also
      Immunization
    physical examination, 1–2
    hepatitis testing in, 2
    needle-stick injuries in, 24–28
      exposure followup, 25f, 26f, 28
      known source, 25, 27–28
      post hepatitis B vaccination,
        26f, 27–28
      unknown source, 24, 25f
    sexually transmitted disease
      testing in, 2
    tuberculosis skin test, in 2
    work status when ill, 4–6
      policy of department, 6
Equipment and supplies
  antishock trousers, 86–87
  CPR manikin, cleaning and
    maintenance, 76–79
  disposable, reuse of, 74, 76
  multidose vials, 79–80
  needle and syringe disposal,
    80–82, 81f, 82f
  respiratory therapy equipment,
    maintenance of, 82–86
    Ambu bag sterilization, 83, 84f
    O_2 humidifiers, 82–83
    suction equipment, 83–86,
      85f, 86f
  stethoscopes, 79
  supply rotation of, 79

Fever blisters. See Herpes
  simplex, oral infection
Fever of unknown origin,
  protective (preventive)
  measures in, 9
Fingers, herpetic whitlow of, 55–
  56, 55f, 97
Flu. See Influenza
Fungus, 101

German measles. See Rubella
Germicidal, 101
Gloves, disposable, when to use,
  10, 11, 95
Glutaraldehyde, for disinfecting
  patient-care equipment,
  66–67t

Gonorrhea, 44–45
  exposure followup, 45
  in pregnant patient, 45
  protective (preventive)
    measures, 45, 96
  symptoms, 44, 45
  transmission, 45, 96

Hand, herpetic whitlow of, 55–56, 55f, 97
Handwashing technique, 11–12
  agents for, 12t
  when to use, 95
Head lice, 51–52
Health status, of EMS personnel, 1–7. *See also* EMS personnel
Hepatitis, 19–28
  A. *See* Hepatitis A
  B. *See* Hepatitis B
  delta agent, 23
  definition of, 101
  needle-stick injuries and, 24–28. *See also* Needle-stick injuries
  non-A, non-B, 23–24
  tests for, in EMS personnel, 2
  toxic, 102
Hepatitis A (viral), 19–20
  in EMS personnel, work status, 5
  exposure followup, 20
  protective (preventive)
    measures, 20, 96
  symptoms, 20
  transmission, 20, 96
Hepatitis B (serum), 20–23
  in dialysis patient, 10
  in EMS personnel, work status, 5
  immunization, 3–4
  protective (preventive)
    measures, 23, 97
  symptoms, 23
  tests for, 2, 21–23, 21t
  transmission, 23, 96
Hepatitis B core antigen, antibody to (anti-HB$_c$), 21t, 22
Hepatitis B immune globulin, for needle-stick injuries, 27
Hepatitis B surface antigen (HB$_s$Ag), 21, 21t
  antibody to (anti-HB$_s$), 21t, 22
Herpes simplex, 53–59
  autoinfection, 59
  genital infection, 56–59
    exposure followup, 59
    female, 57–59, 58f
    male, 56–57, 57f
    in pregnancy, 57–58
    protective (preventive)
      measures, 59, 97
    symptoms, 58–59
    transmission, 58, 97
  in newborn, 57
  oral infection, 54–55, 54f
    in EMS personnel, work status, 5
    exposure followup, 55
    protective (preventive)
      measures, 55, 97
    transmission, 97
  symptoms, 53
  treatment, 59
Herpes viruses, 52–61, 97
  simplex, 53–59
  zoster, 60–61
Herpes zoster (shingles), 60–61
  chickenpox and, 60
  in EMS personnel, work status, 5
  exposure followup, 61
  protective (preventive)
    measures, 61, 97
  transmission, 61, 97
Herpetic whitlow, 55–56, 55f
  in EMS personnel, work status, 5

exposure followup, 56
protective (preventive)
  measures, 56, 97
transmission, 97
Hibiclens, 12t
Hibistat, 12t
Hospital, relations with EMS
  system, 92–94
Hydrophobia. See Rabies

Icterus. See Jaundice
Immune serum globulin (ISG), for
  needle-stick injuries, 24
Immunization, 2–4
  chickenpox (varicella zoster
    immune globulin), 41t
  hepatitis B, 3–4
    for needle-stick injuries, 24
  influenza, 3
  mumps, 3
  rabies, 34
  rubella (German measles), 3
  tetanus-diphtheria, 2
Impetigo, 36
  in EMS personnel, work status, 5
Infection, 102. See also
  Communicable diseases
  airborne, 101
  prevention of, 9–15. See also
    Infection control
  risk to EMS personnel from,
    formula for determining, 6
  signs and symptoms of, 9–11
Infection control, 9–15. See also
  Protective (preventive)
  measures
  cost of program, 89–90
  CPR manikin cleaning and
    maintenance, 76–79, 78f
  handwashing technique, 11–12
  infectious waste disposal, 68–
    69, 70–71, 74t, 75f

IV bags, 87
IV site preparation, 13, 14t, 15f
multidose vials, 79–80
needle and syringe disposal,
  80–82
recognizing signs and
  symptoms, 9–11
record keeping (log sheets), 69–
  70, 70f, 71f, 72–73f
rescue vehicle cleaning and
  disinfection, 65–69
respiratory therapy equipment
  cleaning and maintenance,
  82–86
reuse of disposables, 74, 76
stethoscope cleaning, 79
Infection control practitioner
  (ICP), 92, 94
Infectious wastes
  bagging (packaging) procedures,
    68, 74t
  blood spills, 74, 75f
  definition of, 70
  from peritoneal dialysis patient,
    69
  suction secretions, 84, 85f
Influenza
  in EMS personnel, work status, 5
  immunization, 3
Iodine tincture, for IV site
  preparation, 13, 14t
Isopropyl alcohol, for disinfecting
  rescue vehicle/equipment,
  66t
IV
  bags, 87
  site preparation, 13–15
    antiseptics for, 13, 14t, 15f
    stabilization of needle or
      catheter hub, 13

Jaundice
  definition of, 102

Jaundice (*continued*)
  protective (preventive) measures, 10
Jungle fever. *See* Malaria

Legal liability
  example of, 90
  in reusing disposables, 76
Lice, 51–52, 102
  in EMS personnel, work status, 5
  exposure followup, 52
  protective (preventive) measures, 52, 98
  transmission, 51, 98
Liquid soap antiseptics, for handwashing, 12t
Lockjaw. *See* Tetanus
Log sheets, 69–70
  infection control inquiry form, 72–73f
  infection control procedure form, 70f
  special procedures from, 71f

Malaria (jungel fever), 31–32, 33f
  expsoure followup, 32
  protective (preventive) measures, 32, 98
  symptoms, 31–32
  transmission, 31, 32, 98
Masks, protective, when to use, 9, 95
Measles
  German. *See* Rubella
  red (rubeola), 37–38, 37f
    in EMS personnel, work status, 5
    exposure followup, 38
    protective (preventive) measures, 38, 98
    symptoms, 37, 38
    transmission, 37, 38, 98

Meningitis, 28–31, 102
  aseptic, 30–31
    protective (preventive) measures, 31, 99
    symptoms, 31
    transmission, 31, 99
  bacterial, 29–30
    exposure followup, 30
    protective (preventive) measures, 30, 99
    symptoms, 29, 30
    transmission, 30, 99
  risk to EMS personnel from, application of formula for infection, 7
Meningococcal meningitis, 29–30
Mononucleosis
  definition of, 102
  in EMS personnel, work status, 5
Mumps, 40
  complications, 40
  in EMS personnel, work status, 5
  exposure followup, 40
  immunization, 3
  protective (preventive) measures, 40
  symptoms, 40
  transmission, 40

Needles
  disposal policy and procedure, 80–82, 81f, 82f
  introduction and stabilization of, IV site preparation for, 13, 14t, 15f
Neeldle-stock injuries, 24–28
  exposure followup, 25f, 26f, 28
  known source, 25, 27–28
  post hepatitis B vaccination, 26f, 27–28
  unknown source, 24, 25f
Neisseria meningitiss, 29

Oxygen setups (humidifiers), policy and procedure for use, 82–83

Pediculosis (lice), 51–52
Penicillin, in syphilis, 46
Pertussis (whooping cough), 42–44
  exposure followup, 44
  immunization, 43
  protective (preventive) measured, 44, 99
  symptoms, 42–43
  transmission, 43, 99
Phenol, for disinfecting rescue vehicle/equipment, 67t
Povidone-iodine
  for handwashing, 12t
  for IV site preparation, 13, 14t
PPD (purified protein derivative). See Tuberculosis, screening and testing procedures
Pregnancy
  gonorrhea during, 45
  (genital) herpes during, 57–58
  rubella during, 38
Prepadyne, 12t
Protective (preventive) measures, 95–100
  in AIDS, 49, 50, 95–96
  in aseptic meningitis, 31, 99
  in bacterial meningitis, 30, 99
  in chickenpox, 41, 96
  in cytomegalovirus infection, 51, 96
  in diarrhea, 10
  in fever of unknown origin, 9
  in hepatitis A, 20, 96
  in hepatitis, B, 23, 96
  in herpes simplex
    genital, 59, 97
    herpetic whitlow, 56, 97
    oral, 55, 97
  in herpes zoster, 61, 97
  in impetigo, 36
  in lice, 52, 98
  in malaria, 32, 98
  in measles
    German (rubella), 39, 98
    red (rubeola), 38, 98
  in meningitis, 30, 31, 99
  in pertussis (whooping cough), 44, 99
  in rabies, 34, 99
  in rash, 9
  in salmonella infection, 36, 100
  in scabies, 52, 100
  in syphilis, 46, 100
  in tuberculosis, 17, 99
Pruritus, 102

Quats (quaternary ammonium compounds), for disinfecting rescue vehicle/equipment, 67t

Rabies (hydrophobia), 32, 34, 35t
  exposure followup, 34, 35t
  prophylaxis, 34, 35t
  protective (preventive) measures, 34, 99
  symptoms, 34
  transmission, 32, 34, 99
  treatment, 35t
Rash, protective (preventive) measures in, 9
Record keeping. See Log sheets
Rescue Vehicle
  cleaning and disinfecting, 65–69
    blood spills, 74, 75f
    after communicable disease transport, 68–69
    disinfectants for, 66–67t
    infectious waste disposal, 68–69, 70–71, 74, 74t, 75f

Rescue Vehicle, cleaning and
  disinfecting (*continued*)
  needle and syringe disposal,
    80–82, 81f, 82f
  supply rotation, 79
Red measles. *See* Measles, red
Respiratory infection, upper, in
  EMS personnel, work
  status, 5
Respiratory therapy equipment
  Ambu bag, 83, 84f
  O_2 humidifiers, 82–83
  suction equipment, 83–86, 85f,
    86f
Rubella (German measles), 38–39,
    39f
  exposure followup, 39
  immunization, 3
  during pregnancy, 3
  protective (preventive)
    measures, 39, 98
  symptoms, 38
  transmission, 38–39, 98
Rubeola. *See* Measles, red

Salmonella infection, 34–36
  exposure followup, 36
  protective (preventive)
    measures, 36, 100
  symptoms, 34, 36
  transmission, 35, 36, 100
Scabies, 52, 102
  in EMS personnel, work status,
    5
  exposure followup, 52
  protective (preventive)
    measures, 52, 100
  transmission, 100
Sexually transmitted diseases,
    44–52. *See also specific
    diseases*
  AIDS, 46–50, 95
  cytomegalovirus infection, 50–
    51, 96

gonorrhea, 44–45, 96
herpes, 56–59, 97
lice, 51–52, 98
syphilis, 45–46, 100
tets for, in EMS personnel, 2
Shingles. *See* Herpes zoster
Soaps for handwashing, 12t
Sterility
  of disposable items, 76
  of IV bags, 87
Stethoscope, cleaning, 79
Streptococcal infection, in EMS
  personnel, work status, 5
Suction equipment
  policy and procedure for use,
    83–86, 85f
  cleaning procedure, 84, 86
Supply rotation, 79
Syphilis, 45–46
  exposure followup, 46
  protective (preventive)
    measures, 46, 100
  symptoms, 45–46
  transmission, 100

Tests
  for hepatitis, 2
    type A (viral), 20
    type B (serum), 21–22, 21t
  for sexually transmitted
    diseases, in EMS personnel
    2
  for tuberculosis, 2, 17, 18t
Tetanus
  definition of, 102
  immunization, 2
Toxicity, of disposable items,
    76
Tuberculosis, 16–19
  in EMS personnel, work
    status, 4
  exposure followup, 17, 19
  protective (preventive)
    measures, 17, 99

screening and testing procedures, 2, 18f
symptoms, 17
transmission, 17, 99

Vaccination. *See* Immunization
Vaccine, 103
Varicella (chickenpox), 40–42, 42f
Varicella zoster immune globulin, exposure criteria for use of, 41t
Viricidal, 103

Waste materials. *See* Infectious waste
Whooping cough. *See* Pertussis
Workers Compensation, in needle-stock injuries, 28
Wounds, draining
in EMS personnel, work status, 5
in patient, protective (preventive) measures, 10